Visiting the Memory Café
and other Dementia Care Activities

by the same author

**Developing Excellent Care for People Living
with Dementia in Care Homes**
Caroline Baker
Foreword by Professor Murna Downs
ISBN 978 1 84905 467 6
eISBN 978 1 78450 053 5

of related interest

Doll Therapy in Dementia Care
Evidence and Practice
Gary Mitchell
Foreword by Sally Knocker
ISBN 978 1 84905 570 3
eISBN 978 1 78450 007 8

Facilitating Spiritual Reminiscence for People with Dementia
A Learning Guide
Elizabeth MacKinlay and Corinne Trevitt
ISBN 978 1 84905 573 4
eISBN 978 1 78450 018 4

A Creative Toolkit for Communication in Dementia Care
Karrie Marshall
ISBN 978 1 84905 694 6
eISBN 978 1 78450 206 5

Activities for Older People in Care Homes
A Handbook for Successful Activity Planning
Sarah Crockett
ISBN 978 1 84905 429 4
eISBN 978 0 85700 839 8

Visiting the
Memory Café

and other
Dementia Care Activities

*Evidence-based Interventions
for Care Homes*

EDITED BY CAROLINE BAKER *and*
JASON CORRIGAN-CHARLESWORTH

FOREWORD BY DR G. ALLEN POWER

Jessica Kingsley *Publishers*
London and Philadelphia

First published in 2017
by Jessica Kingsley Publishers
73 Collier Street
London N1 9BE, UK
and
400 Market Street, Suite 400
Philadelphia, PA 19106, USA

www.jkp.com

Library of Congress Cataloging in Publication Data
A CIP catalog record for this book is available from the Library of Congress

British Library Cataloguing in Publication Data
A CIP catalogue record for this book is available from the British Library

ISBN 978 1 78592 252 7
eISBN 978 1 78450 535 6

Printed and bound in the United States

This book is dedicated to all of our residents living with dementia, their relatives and the amazing staff who look after them so well.

Any proceeds from the sale of the book will be donated to Barchester's Charitable Foundation, which is a registered charity that helps older people and other adults with a disability living within the community across England, Scotland and Wales.

www.bhcfoundation.org.uk

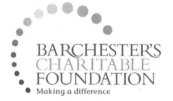

BARCHESTER'S
CHARITABLE
FOUNDATION
Making a difference

Contents

Foreword

Nearly 300,000 people are living with dementia in residential care homes across the UK, and millions more worldwide. While such communities strive to provide optimal care and support, many people living with the diagnosis experience various types of distress, some quite frequently; and many are medicated with potentially harmful psychoactive medications as a result.

In my work to help eliminate the use of such harmful medications, I have learned that the drugs themselves are not the real problem. They are only a symptom of a care system that does not understand how to support the well-being of those living in their communities. Part of this misunderstanding stems from a misguided view that the person's distress is primarily the result of brain disease (often termed 'behavioural and psychological symptoms of dementia'); part of the misunderstanding also results from viewing our role narrowly as providing housing, medical support, and personal care, while failing to recognise other life-giving needs that make every person want to get out of bed in the morning.

The well-being model referenced in this book is my adaptation of a framework developed in a 2005 white paper[1] that was supported by a grant from The Eden Alternative®, an

---

1 Re-released as The Eden Alternative Domains of Well-Being™: Revolutionizing the experience of home by bringing well-being to life. Available at http://www.edenalt.org/wordpress/wp-content/uploads/2014/02/Eden AltWellBeingWhitePaperv5.f.

international non-profit organisation 'dedicated to creating quality of life for elders and their care partners, wherever they may live'. In that paper, the authors identified seven 'domains' of well-being that they felt were applicable to people of all ages, cultures, and abilities. The paper contends that these essential aspects of a life worth living are too often underappreciated, even ignored in most aged care settings.

In an effort to find a better approach, I adapted and re-ordered those seven domains as follows: identity, connectedness, security, autonomy, meaning, growth, and joy, exploring how each domain is challenged (by the illness and by our care systems), and showing how a transformational model can greatly improve the lives of people living with a diagnosis of dementia.

What is revealed is that the erosion of various aspects of well-being is the root cause of most of the distress we are currently medicating; and a quick glance at the seven domains listed above should make it abundantly clear why pills cannot solve the problem. What does work, however, is an appreciative approach that works proactively to enhance each of these seven domains for each individual, thus removing the root cause of most of the distress people experience, and creating more sustainable success, without harmful medications.

The team at Barchester Healthcare has taken this concept to heart, using the well-being framework to design, implement, and evaluate the various programmes they offer for those living with dementia, and gradually introducing them in over 160 aged care communities across the UK. Each chapter of this book describes the successes and challenges of the various approaches, and shows how they fulfill each well-being domain.

Throughout the book, the team presents a wealth of qualitative and narrative information; in doing so, they also provide a roadmap for other organisations who might wish to try similar approaches, but who may lack the resources and expertise to conduct formal research on their efforts. The chapters are practical, compelling, and highly readable.

Most important, however, is that the Barchester team has broken free of the traditional paradigms of 'managing challenging behaviours' or offering generic, one-size-fits-all programming solutions that fail to meet individual needs and desires. So this book is also a roadmap for organisations to transform the underpinnings of their initiatives—from a narrow institutional view of 'care' to a mindset with the flexibility to identify and respond to each person's needs and preferences, and to create the soil in which people living with dementia can flourish to the fullest extent possible.

Just as each initiative is measured against the well-being model, the seven domains provide a useful guide to help understand what is necessary for a truly individualised, relational approach. First, the domain of identity reminds us of the uniqueness of every individual, regardless of her diagnosis—a uniqueness that, if anything, becomes more striking as a person lives with dementia, because each individual will respond to the cognitive changes in a manner dictated by her unique history and personal attributes. Connectedness tells us that the only way to nourish an optimal sense of well-being is through close, continuous relationships that topple the walls of professional distance to enable deep caring and empathy.

Moving to the next two domains of security and autonomy, we see the need to develop a sense of trust, dignity, and respect between ourselves and those we support, and to use our deep knowing to negotiate risk and enable choice in as safe a manner as possible. We learn that in order for life to have meaning, people must continue to have purposeful roles, even when living in residential care, and that we must strive to find ways for people to visibly contribute to the life of the community as far as they are able. It is only through authentic relationships and truly meaningful living that personal growth can occur; and with proper support, such growth is possible throughout people's lives with dementia.

Lastly, we understand that well-being is not simply the absence of all distress; in fact, our expectations for people living with dementia far exceed what we demand of ourselves with respect to our ability to experience times of anger, frustration, or sadness. The concept of joy is much more than simply being happy. It means creating a deep sense of personal and spiritual fulfillment that sustains people through good times and bad, with the support of the authentic relationships developed within the community.

In summary, Visiting the Memory Café is much more than a roster of programs and therapies; it is a guide to a new way of thinking about how to best serve the individuals in our communities, and it provides a framework for evaluating whether your approaches support the people in your care to the fullest extent. I hope that as you explore this book, you will be inspired to think of ways in which your own organisation can shift from simply mitigating decline to creating true well-being for all of the members of your community.

G. Allen Power, MD

Rochester, New York, USA

10 July 2017

Acknowledgements

The people that we need to thank first and foremost are our wonderful residents living in our Memory Lane Communities within the organisation. Thank you for letting us try out our new activities with you; we are really pleased that most of them have been (and continue to be) a big hit!

Second, we would like to thank our amazing relatives and friends for helping to provide us with life story information, favourite music, photographs and memorabilia, and for your support with our programme.

Third, we would like to give a special mention to the fantastic staff working within the care homes. Your dedication, enthusiasm and levels of person-centred care for people living with dementia are a joy to observe.

We would also like to thank our team – a collection of dementia care specialists (who all have chapters in this book) – for always 'going the extra mile' to ensure that our residents, relatives and staff within the homes are fully supported across the UK.

Furthermore, the new dementia care programme would not have been possible without the full support, encouragement and guidance of our board of directors and senior management team at Barchester Healthcare, who have helped us not only to build a great team, but also to roll this programme out across all 160 care homes, providing care for people living with dementia.

We would also like to extend a particular thank-you to Sara Jones, Namaste project worker with St Luke's Cheshire Hospice/The End of Life Partnership, for working alongside the team at Adlington Manor Care Home to help to improve the lives and well-being of residents living with advanced dementia.

Our colleagues in the marketing department have been such a help to us in getting the Getting to Know Me Board Game and Book professionally produced, and our colleagues across the company have all been so supportive of the programme and helped us to get it off the ground.

Last but not least, we are extremely grateful to the team at Jessica Kingsley Publishers who have helped us to put this collection of activities and interventions together as readable chapters!

The Contributors

Caroline Baker

Beginning as a care assistant on a dementia care ward, Caroline went on to qualify as a Registered Mental Nurse (RMN) in 1989 and is now the Director of Dementia Care at Barchester Healthcare, working with a team of seven specialists to support over 160 care homes that care for people living with dementia. Caroline won a Lifetime Achievement Award in Dementia Care in 2014 and is the author of *Developing Excellent Care for People Living with Dementia in Care Homes* (2014; Jessica Kingsley Publishers). Caroline has recently worked alongside the team to develop a new programme of dementia care delivery to enhance dementia care, called 10-60-06, which has achieved some incredible outcomes for people living with dementia.

Jason Corrigan-Charlesworth

Jason has worked in a caring role for people living with dementia for nearly 30 years, undertaking various roles within different organisations in this time. He initially commenced his career as a care assistant and worked his way up to be a home manager and then a regional manager. Jason then decided to put his skills and knowledge into training and development and for the past 15 years has specialised in dementia care, ensuring that those providing care delivery do so in a person-centred, holistic manner. Jason's current role as Deputy Director of Dementia Care reflects this passion and dedication in improving the quality of life not only for people living with dementia, but also for those who care for them.

Ann Marie Harmer

Ann Marie qualified as a nurse in 1987 and has worked within Barchester Healthcare for over ten years as a dementia care specialist. Ann Marie is currently undertaking an MSc in Dementia Care and was a finalist in 2016 for the UK Dementia Congress (UKDC) awards for developing the Getting to Know Me Board Game. Ann Marie has a real commitment to ensuring that people living with dementia receive the very best of care, and currently works within the central region of Barchester Healthcare helping to support a number of care homes.

Phil Harper

Phil's career in nursing spans a period of 45 years. During the later years of his professional life Phil specialised in elderly care and is now dedicated to dementia care development both for people living with dementia and their carers. Following 40 years of working in the NHS, his present role as a dementia care specialist allows him to share his knowledge and experience of dementia care with others. Phil admits that caring for people living with dementia can at times be difficult but to specialise in this career is an extremely rewarding life experience.

Deena Heaney

Deena is a dementia care specialist working as part of the dementia team at Barchester Healthcare. Deena has worked in various roles within the private sector over the past 30 years. A three-time care award winner, Deena has a recognised teaching qualification and has developed and delivered exceptional training packages, supporting staff teams in enhancing the wellbeing of residents living with dementia.

David Owen

David Owen is currently a dementia care specialist with Barchester Healthcare. He has worked for Barchester for 15 years. His background has foundations as a qualified nurse for over 30 years, working within many roles and responsibilities in the NHS, and private and voluntary sectors of the health industy. He also has qualifications and an interest in talking therapies. His connections with dementia are personal and professional, with a close school friend living with Huntington's disease, and close family members also part of his experience. This experience along with his own health challenges have driven his passion and commitment to developing dementia services and mental health services. The dementia experience, he believes, is always more colourful and positive for an individual who goes into care where family-like relationships are built between residents, family and staff.

Claire Peart

Claire has worked within the care industry since leaving school, initially as a healthcare assistant, and then enrolling as a student nurse in 1992. Since qualifying as a nurse over 20 years ago she has worked in various roles in elderly care within the private sector for a number of different organisations, including as head of a complex dementia unit in North East England. Claire has a keen interest in the implementation of music therapy and technological interventions to support people living with dementia. She currently works as a dementia care specialist for Barchester

Healthcare, supporting care homes throughout Scotland, and North East and North West England.

Holly Rance

Holly Rance started her career in interior design with a Bachelor of Arts Degree in Interior Design from the University of Bournemouth. She then went on to work for various design consultancies specialising in residential interiors, hotels and high-end furniture and yacht design. Holly has worked within the care sector for the past 7 years and has re-developed the aesthetic and brand identity of one of the country's largest care groups. The proven success of this has naturally led on to her creating a dementia concept in conjunction with dementia specialists to develop an environment that is unique and calm, and will enhance the lives of the residents who live in the homes. Holly is passionate about design; her love for creating not only beautiful interiors but ones that are functional and practical is her fundamental approach to design and life.

Leon Smith

Leon has worked within the care industry for just over 25 years; he started out as a carer looking after people with learning disabilities and sensory impairments. He has worked in and managed many different types of care services including a home for people recovering from drug and alcohol dependency, a care home for deaf-blind people, as well as various residential services for the elderly. Leon has always returned to his passion, which is the care of people living with dementia. He has been working as a dementia care specialist for several years and enjoys supporting our homes to offer the highest possible specialist dementia care for our residents, their families and the staff teams.

Introduction

CAROLINE BAKER

From the moment of birth, we are encouraged by others to engage in activity that will provide fun, education, social interaction or individual engagement of the senses. As a baby this may involve a game of 'peek-a-boo', singing lullabies, shaking a rattle or reading a book to entertain, provide comfort or to encourage rest. In our childhood years, we are persuaded to take part in physical activities and sports days, promoting our competitive edge. But we are also exposed to social activity where we learn to make friends and get along with each other; often activities are chosen for us and we have to comply. As we move into adulthood, our choice to be involved in activity becomes less pressured (with the exception of peer pressure!) and our true choice of the things that we wish to be engaged in or actively involved in becomes shaped by our own interests and those aspects that we deem would improve our own well-being, be that physically, psychologically, socially or spiritually. For some of us, activity is high on the agenda. For others, engagement rather than activity is key.

Along with the general view of 'activity', we also all have a role in life (if not several) and part of the function of that role is to fulfil a need for ourselves if not also fulfilling a need for others. Whether that role is a mother, father, sister, employer, employee or a member of the crown green bowling club, we generally carry out our roles as well as we can to maintain our own well-being. The point we are making here is…why should everything stop if somebody moves into a care home?

10-60-06 dementia care programme

The organisation we work for has just over 200 care homes, 160 of which provide care for people living with dementia in specialist units, called Memory Lane Communities. As a relatively new team of eight dementia care specialists, we really wanted to find a way that we could help staff to deliver the latest evidenced and research-based practices within the care homes and also to implement some of our own ideas that we thought may help in relation to activity provision.

Our starting point was our new mission statement, which led our 10-60-06 programme to have a real focus on activity or engagement for the person living with dementia,

People living with dementia are admitted into our care homes on various stages of their journey, but whichever path they are on in the complex map of cognitive impairment, we need to prioritise the reduction of any distress and the promotion of their well-being.

Our approach underpinning Memory Lane is to help the residents in our care to continue their lives as independently as possible by working alongside them rather than for them and by promoting positive memories wherever we can.

The person is our focus rather than the diagnosis, and when we do this, it allows us to work with the resident in a natural way without preconceptions.

Our staff will be skilled in dementia care interventions and will be chosen for their empathic approach towards people living with dementia.

Our environments will reduce confusion and promote orientation as well as offering evidenced and research-based interventions to assist our residents to achieve fulfilment in our homes.

The 10-60-06 programme itself involves a number of evidence- or research-based criteria that the homes need to implement, along with four levels of training,[2] but during the pilot phase (across 12 homes) we also decided to implement a number of new activities that had not previously been evaluated by the organisation. During team discussions around which activities we would try, some members of the team initiated their own ideas, which transpired in some amazing activities that had incredible outcomes for the residents involved. The programme and the team (and individuals within the team) reached the finals for six awards last year and we have delivered presentations in the UK, Budapest and Oslo, and in July 2017 will deliver a presentation at the Pioneer Network Conference in Chicago.

This book explores a range of activities that have either been developed by the team or introduced by the team to enhance dementia care within the care home environment, but many of the ideas could also be introduced within any community setting or the person's own home. The book is a real team effort (each team member contributing at least one chapter) and has evolved as a result of the new programme.

Seven domains of well-being

Throughout the book, you will see that most of the chapters refer to the seven domains of well-being and how the

---

2   The term 10-60-06 derives from the number of criteria within each section. The first 10 criteria apply across the whole home and are key to delivering person centred care. The next 60 criteria apply to the more specialist interventions in dementia care and the last 6 criteria apply to interventions that were tried and tested in the original pilot programme and have been taken forward for all homes now undertaking the programme.

particular activities relate to the seven domains. Our training and the observational tool that we have developed centre around the domains which were adapted and developed by Al Power (2014), a geriatrician based in the USA who is absolutely passionate about the needs of people living with dementia and is highly acclaimed internationally because of the extent of his knowledge and its applicability to changing the culture of dementia care.

What do people living with dementia tell us?

Dementia is more prevalent in older people, and this can often be accompanied by other health issues, including mental health conditions such as depression (Department of Health (DOH) 2016). So if we hope to enhance overall well-being, we need to be mindful to address not only the person's physiological symptoms but also their psychological, sociological and spiritual needs, and thus we can begin to enhance all four areas through a range of activities or interventions that the resident may enjoy.

However, we also need to be mindful that activities really need to be tailored for the person living with dementia and that we don't bring an individual into a large group of people if that is not something that the person has enjoyed in the past. We also need to be acutely aware that within a care home environment specifically, activities are not the responsibility of the lead co-ordinator but the responsibility of us all. Potentially, everything we do can become a meaningful activity.

Within her book, Kate Swaffer (2016) states that being diagnosed with dementia, and living with the symptoms of dementia, are definitely not as much fun as having a birthday party, but having dementia is no reason to give up living or to 'die' straight away. Often the perception of many outside of the direct care field is that care homes are a place of 'no hope and no future', particularly if you have a diagnosis of dementia, but we have seen high levels of well-being for people living within our homes because we encourage people to be as involved as they are able (or want to).

I am sure that Kate is not referring to specifically providing a range of meaningful activities to fulfil her needs, but perhaps she is telling us that it remains hugely important to have a sense of meaning in her life following her diagnosis. Kate has been a true ambassador for people living with dementia and has spoken at many conferences and has written several publications and blogs. These particular activities for Kate, it seems, are providing her with strength, ambition and recognition.

However, preferences for involvement or engagement in activity are very different for every individual; some may prefer 'doing', and others may prefer to observe but still remain engaged rather than involved.

Christine Bryden (2005) informs us that, 'With the stress of many activities at once, I become very focused, trying with all the brain I have left to concentrate. Telling me to rest won't help, but helping me to complete the task will.' She goes on to say that the most important factor for improving care is the environment, as this can be changed quite easily to ensure that it enhances the person's sense of safety, value and well-being. She elaborates further by informing the reader that it needs to validate the person's experiences and emotions, facilitate the person's actions, celebrate the person's abilities and provide sensory pleasures.

Content

It is helpful to read Chapter 1 before the other chapters, as the subject of this chapter – getting to know our residents really well – underpins everything we do in dementia care. Other than that, feel free to dip in and out of any chapter.

In Chapter 1, Ann Marie Harmer talks about two new life story activities that have been developed by her and her colleague, David Owen, which have since been professionally produced and rolled out across the organisation. The first is a book called 'Getting to Know Me' that helps residents to document the key memories that can be shared with staff to help them to deliver person-centred care. The second is a board game, also called 'Getting to Know Me', that staff can play with the residents to obtain the information to complete the book with them.

In Chapter 2, the readers are introduced to an intervention designed and developed by the author, Claire Peart, which encompasses a digital approach to reminiscence therapy. Rolling slide shows categorised into either the 1950s or the 1960s are picture shows with accompanying music and text which are placed predominately in 'rest areas' within the corridor. The slide shows have had a phenomenal impact on some of the residents within our care homes, so much so that although this intervention was originally only intended for the homes that Claire was working with, it was also implemented into many of the other pilot homes.

In Chapter 3, David Owen explores the use of the Namaste approach in care homes and how the use of Namaste has helped to improve well-being and increased nutrition within the care home. Namaste Care involves a blend of sensory approaches and is carried out with a small group of residents in a dedicated area. The Namaste programme is carried out for two hours each morning and afternoon over a seven-day period, with staff receiving training in sensory activities. The staff working within the home have really enjoyed being involved in delivering Namaste Care and again, this will also be delivered in many other of our care homes as we roll the programme out.

In Chapter 4, Jason Corrigan-Charlesworth talks about the implementation of empathy dolls within the care home setting and how their use has really helped the residents to engage, reminisce and improve their well-being. There is much more written about the use of doll therapy now but it was so important within our programme that we just couldn't leave it out!

In Chapter 5, Jason Corrigan-Charlesworth's second chapter, he talks about the implementation of Memory Cafés within the care home setting. Sometimes hard to implement and maintain, Memory Cafés can be incredibly helpful not only to those living with dementia but also to the families and friends who may want to find out more about dementia or simply to gather support from others living with the condition or supporting those who do.

In Chapter 6, Phil Harper shares with us the insights and observations he made when introducing programmes of physical activity into several care homes for people living with dementia. Having witnessed one of these sessions when accrediting a home, I could clearly see the joy and laughter as residents (and relatives) engaged in the sessions.

In Chapter 7, Leon Smith shares a story of something that we have not often seen used in dementia care. His chapter focuses on guided imagery accompanied by smells, sounds and sometimes visual images to help residents to relax, draw on their memories and chatter to each other about their experiences.

In Chapter 8, Deena Heaney talks about the importance of maintaining daily living skills and how these can be incorporated into everyday life in the care home, helping people to maintain a sense of purpose and increase their well-being. Some of our residents simply want to relax when they come into our care homes but, for others, keeping busy is really important to maintain their self-esteem.

In Chapter 9, Caroline Baker and Holly Rance write about the importance of the environment in enhancing dementia care. Often our residents are transferred from hospitals where they may already have had several transfers (of wards or bays) and we need to ensure that we try to reduce any further confusion or frustration as much as we can. Additionally, we aim to provide engagement on the journey for people who wish to walk around and places where they may stay and rest.

In Chapter 10, Caroline Baker will summarise the results of the programme and discuss further interventions or activities that were implemented to enhance well-being.

Although we were confident at the beginning of the programme that some of the interventions or activities would make a difference, we have been absolutely delighted with the results that they have brought: so much so, that we felt we had to share them with you all. Anybody who works in dementia care really only has one major goal, and that is to improve the lives of people living with dementia; so it is only fair that if we have found something that works well, we share best practice.

We all really hope that you enjoy reading about this collection of activities that we have tried and tested.

Please note that names have been changed throughout the book to protect the identity of service users and care staff.

1

The Importance of Getting to Know *Me*

ANN MARIE HARMER

In this chapter I will explore how recognising and understanding individuals' life stories is the key to personalising their care. This chapter will describe a board game that has created an innovative means of exploring and identifying the values, beliefs and habits that have shaped individuals' lives. This chapter will also describe how the information and knowledge gained from playing the game is transferred into a unique life story booklet.

The year 1987 was the start of my career in caring for individuals living with dementia. Reality orientation was widely used to support individuals who had a diagnosis of dementia (Jones and Miesen 1996). This approach endeavoured to help those experiencing dementia to be aware of where they were and what was happening to them. It was later identified that this technique remained useful for individuals living in the earlier stage of dementia but caused distress to those further along in their journey living with dementia (Baker 2015).

On one occasion I remember using the reality orientation technique when I saw a lady, living with dementia, stroking her reflection in a mirror. As she was doing so, she was smiling and saying, 'Mum, Mum.' Just as I had been trained to do I said, 'That's not your mum, that is you.' At that moment I felt that I had broken that lady's heart. I felt that I had taken away the comfort and happiness she had experienced seeing her mother. Potentially I had also taken away years of her life: she had not recognised herself as an older person as in her reality she was much younger. I would never consider using this technique in a similar situation today. Now I would respond by acknowledging the person's reality by using validation therapy and saying, 'I imagine your mum is a lovely lady.' Baker (2015) described validation therapy as a means of recognising and working alongside the individual's reality.

On another occasion I assumed that all the residents wanted to watch and mark the Remembrance Day service at the Cenotaph in Whitehall. The care team and I set the lounge chairs around the television and each resident had a poppy to wear. The majority of the residents appeared to be engaged watching the television and some joined in with the hymns being sung. All was going well until the bugler played the last post. Harry immediately stood up and screamed, 'No, no, no!' He threw his cup onto the floor, pushed an empty chair over and marched around the unit shouting, 'No, no, no!' When I explained to Harry's wife what had happened she shared that Harry had taken part in the World War II battle of Arnhem. It transpired that this battle was where Harry's brother and friends had been killed. Harry had stood beside each of their graves to the sound of a bugler playing the last post. My assumption that everyone would want to watch the Remembrance service and not knowing Harry's life story resulted in Harry experiencing severe distress. If I had known what Harry had endured in his life I would never have introduced him to anything that would make him relive such distressing memories. That was the moment that I recognised the importance of knowing and recognising the life stories and emotional memories of people living with dementia.

In order for caregivers to truly deliver person-centred care they need to know where individuals have come from, what they have experienced and their emotional memories. Having this information also helps caregivers recognise individuals' experiences of dementia, their needs and their responses. This information also gives caregivers clues to the true meanings behind the words and responses which at first can appear baffling or meaningless. When people's values, beliefs and habits that have shaped their lives are fully understood, recognised and respected it is then that caregivers are enabled to personalise the care of people living with dementia.

In 2006 my dear Aunt Vi began her journey living with dementia. She was living in the same assisted living complex as my mum. For a long time both Mum and Aunt Vi had their own routine in sharing the cooking of meals but, as time passed, each time it was Aunt Vi's turn to cook she chose to buy them both a take-away meal. We had not recognised it at the time but Aunt Vi had been trying to hide that she was experiencing difficulty in completing certain tasks. I was alerted that Aunt Vi was experiencing some challenges when she was unable to count her money to pay for items, and although her handbag was often heavy with loose change, she would hand over notes to the cashiers. Aunt Vi would say to me, 'I'm going daft,' 'I am losing my marbles,' and began walking around the complex turning on lights and knocking on people's doors at night. Aunt Vi was assessed and given a diagnosis of Alzheimer's disease. She agreed to move into one of our care homes for four weeks for further assessment. Before Aunt Vi moved into the home I wrote her life story and made a memory book with photos of her family, pets and favourite places.

Photos are invaluable in person-centred dementia care. Photos of the person when they were much younger can often remind caregivers that the residents were once just like us, with busy lives and families. One photo in Aunt Vi's memory book shows Aunt Vi cleaning Princess Diana's wedding dress following the Royal Wedding. This photo is a key to relieving any distress Aunt Vi may experience. Her attention could easily be diverted from what had upset her to talking fondly about the Royal family and of her pressing and cleaning all the royal clothes.

As I worked for the company, as a dementia care specialist I wrote Aunt Vi's care plans for the team. In her night-time/sleeping care plan I wrote that when Aunt Vi went to bed she would need a bedside lamp, her torch, her ticking clock, a glass of water, her radio on a talking station such as LBC (Leading Britain's Conversation) and her bedroom curtains not fully closed. The reasons behind these requirements were that during World War II Aunt Vi had become trapped alone in the dark coal cellar. She was also trapped on two occasions in the London Underground. The first time was the Moorgate tube crash in 1975 and the second was the King's Cross fire in 1987. Aunt Vi was terrified of being alone in the dark. This could provide some explanation as to why she turned on all the lights and knocked on doors in the assisted living complex where she lived.

I documented Aunt Vi's emotional memories and explained that if they showed her the Royal family books she had in her bedroom, she would happily talk about the Royal family. Aunt Vi had been to Buckingham Palace and had pressed the clothes of the Royalty for most of her working life. She had even cleaned and pressed Princess Diana's wedding dress and Prince William's christening gown. Having all this information on Aunt Vi proved invaluable for the team caring for her. This information also enabled the team to understand, recognise and deliver all of Aunt Vi's seven domains of well-being, as described by Power (2014).

Christine Bryden (2016) questioned what meaning individuals have to their lives following a diagnosis of dementia and how others can support people living with dementia to find a meaning to their lives. Bryden described how people living with dementia can be empowered to find meaning in their lives through following Power's (2014) seven domains of well-being:

1. identity

2. connectedness

3. security

4. autonomy

5. meaning

6. growth

7. joy.

How life story work enhances the well-being of people living with dementia

As human beings we all require not only our physical needs to be met but also our psychological, sociological and spiritual needs. The meeting of our psychological needs can help to provide fulfilment, self-actualisation and meaningfulness to our lives. This does not change when a person is living with dementia. The only difference is that the person who has dementia often relies on others to recognise, protect and respect their needs.

Knowing a person's life story equips caregivers with the tools, knowledge and understanding to support the person to live well with dementia.

Identity

When we look at identity, we need to think about our individuality, our sense of wholeness, and having a history that includes a multitude of unique life experiences and emotional memories. We also need to fully understand an individual's life story as an essential key to helping individuals maintain their own personal identity. If we think back to Aunt Vi, showing her the photograph of the wedding dress helped her to remember her work, how much she enjoyed it and all the famous people she met.

Despite being a daughter and wife, Aunt Vi's core role, throughout her life, was that of being an aunt to many nieces and nephews. When she moved into the care home she was asked how she would like to be addressed and she replied, 'Vi'. Within a month I noticed that all the staff were calling her Aunt Vi. A senior carer had identified that when they needed to assist her with transfers using a hoist or assisting her with personal care she would become tense and anxious despite reassuring her. Observing the close relationship between myself and my aunt, the senior carer referred to her as Aunt Vi during personal care. It was then that they witnessed that she became immediately relaxed. By calling her Aunt Vi it enabled her to feel recognised, safe, belonging and connected to her carers. This also evidenced that Aunt Vi's own individual uniqueness had been recognised and respected. Her identity, personality and individuality had been preserved and she was not being treated as part of a group of people living with dementia in a care home.

On one occasion I was sitting with a lady living with early-onset Alzheimer's, and together we looked at her Getting to Know Me Book©. I asked her if she preferred to be called Samantha or Sam. She told me that she preferred to be called by her family nickname for her, which was Fred. This information was recorded in Fred's Getting to Know Me Book and shared with the care team. Discovering this information not only recognised and protected Fred's identity but also created a means of meaningfully connecting with Fred.

Connectedness

As human beings we are a social species with a need to be connected to others, especially in times of experiencing distress and change. Connectedness is a sense of belonging and bonding with a place, other people and personal possessions. People are connected to their past, present and their future. Through understanding individuals' life stories caregivers are enabled to maintain those connections and relationships. When people move into a care home their connections with their own home are often severed and new connections need to be created within their new home. Through the experiences of living with dementia and moving into a care home a person can feel frightened, anxious and embarrassed. This can result in people withdrawing and isolating themselves. Playing the Getting to Know Me Board Game© creates the opportunity to connect with each other in a fun and non-threatening way. Through playing the game and completing the book, discoveries can be made about what is important to people. Through supporting people to maintain relationships with family and friends it can enable those people living with dementia to retain their sense of self.

As family members we nicknamed Aunt Vi the 'Bag Lady'. Aunt Vi was never seen without a bag. When Aunt Vi began her journey living with dementia the bag became increasingly important to her and she would spend a long time rummaging through her shopping bag. When her mobility became a little unstable she brought a four-wheeled shopping trolley that contained her handbag and her shopping. When Aunt Vi moved into the care home, the staff reported that she was walking around the Memory Lane Community (the dementia care unit) collecting various items and putting them into her four-wheeled trolley. They even reported to me that when Aunt Vi went on a trip to a fish and chip restaurant she put her plate into her shopping bag.

After she retired from work Aunt Vi kept herself active. Every day both my mum and Aunt Vi would walk around Hertford town with their four-wheeled trolleys chatting to people they met and doing their shopping. Knowing this information enabled the care team to understand Aunt Vi's reality and behaviour. When Aunt Vi was collecting items around the Memory Lane Community in her reality she was probably shopping. The team did not stop her from doing this but just put items discreetly back to where they belonged. The activity of collecting these items was part of who Aunt Vi was and it was her way of connecting with her environment. It also gave Aunt Vi meaning and purpose to her day and helped her to feel safe and secure. In a strange and unfamiliar environment the activity of collecting items helped Aunt Vi make sense of her day, giving her connectedness, security and control.

Security

There is a need for all of us to feel safe and free from uncertainty, anxiety and fear. Security is more than feeling safe behind coded entrance and exit doors in a dementia community in a care home. Security is about feeling safe in the environment in which we live and with those people we share our homes with. There is a need for everyone to feel both physically and emotionally safe. When a person is living in an unfamiliar environment the cognitive abilities of a person living with dementia might reduce, but their emotions can be enhanced. Knowing Aunt Vi's life story enables the care team to recognise when she becomes overwhelmed by her emotional memories, leading to her experiencing distress. The recognition and understanding of Aunt Vi's life story also equips the care team with the knowledge to distract her to a subject or activity that she enjoys.

Autonomy

Autonomy outlines how people can be given support and opportunities to make choices and have control of their daily life plans and care. Many of us fear losing our independence, and playing the Getting to Know Me Board Game creates the opportunity to discover people's fears, what people can still do and how the care team can support the residents to retain their independence for as long as possible. The person's strengths and abilities can be recorded in their plan of care but also in their Getting to Know Me Book, which was created by David Owen, dementia care specialist with Barchester Healthcare, and author of Chapter 3, to accompany the board game. Where the resident is able, they can also add to the book, sharing their positive memories.

Meaning

People living with dementia need activities that are meaningful, make sense to them and give them a sense of purpose in their lives. Knowing a person's life story can help caregivers offer activities that support the individuality of each resident and enhance their sense of being needed, as well as their self-esteem.

Frank was living with vascular dementia and had been a farmer. He believed that the care team were his farm hands. Each morning Frank would wake early and became anxious to go out and bring his cows in from the fields. In recognising Frank's feeling and to relieve his distress, each morning the care team would tell him that they had milked the cows and they were back in the fields. Frank was reassured with this response and contented enough to sit and eat his breakfast. Some people would argue that this is lying to the person with dementia. I describe this as not lying but entering the person's reality and telling what I would call a 'fiblet': an untruth that supports the individual's well-being. Frank was happy with the statement.

However, in the late afternoon Frank became restless and anxious. The care team found it difficult to understand and recognise what was causing Frank's distress. Following a conversation with Frank's family the team discovered that in the afternoons Frank used to collect eggs to sell in his farm shop. Frank's family brought the basket Frank used to collect eggs. The basket was left by the door into the garden. The care team hid eggs in the garden. Each day Frank would go into the garden and search for eggs to put into his basket. This activity was meaningful to Frank and he no longer showed signs of distress in the afternoons.

Growth

Christine Bryden (2016) stated that when diagnosed with dementia people were faced with a new future ahead of them. Within the care home the care team can support and assist people living with dementia to adjust to the changes within and around them. Being offered opportunities to try new activities and experiences supports and encourages people to live a new life and adapt to living in the moment without judgement, labels and former prejudices. Two of the activities that have proved successful in some care homes are tai chi and Zumba classes. People living in the care homes have described these activities as fun and gentle. Photographs and descriptions of people participating in old and new activities can be recorded in the back of the Getting to Know Me Book. In doing so it supports and reassures relatives that memories continue to be made and that their loved one has fun within their home. This can also help to ease some of the guilt relatives feel when they have had to make the difficult decision of placing their loved one in a care home. The photos and descriptions of the residents participating in activities evidences that people can live well with dementia. The Getting to Know Me Book is not all about finding out about the past; it is also about recording the here and now and any wishes or hopes for the future.

Joy

Christine Bryden (2016) described joy as being one of the most challenging of the seven domains to be achieved. Only when all of the other six domains are sustained will people's well-being be achieved and result in people feeling happy and contented and having a sense of joy in their lives.

People living with dementia can find it very difficult to remember recent events (short-term memory), but many find it easier to clearly recall events they have done years ago (long-term memory). Imagine a filing-cabinet drawer. The back of the drawer represents the day we were born. From that day we are filling the drawer with files containing memories of our experiences and the emotions linked to those many experiences. We continue filling the drawer up until the present day, which is the front of the drawer. If we were diagnosed with dementia the most recent files at the front of the drawer begin to be taken out, and thus our most recent memories are lost. Files for the last 20 years may be taken out and those memories lost forever. This would mean that the person's reality would be that of 20 years ago. By knowing people's life stories caregivers are assisted to recognise what the individuals' reality is and know how to support them in their reality.

The Getting to Know Me Book

The process of discovering a person's life story enables staff to connect and build positive relationships with individuals living with dementia and their families and friends. The Getting to Know Me Book was developed to support the creation of positive moments within dementia care communities by sharing memories, likes and dislikes. Information gained supports the maintaining of people's identity through all aspects of their dementia journey. The book works in parallel with the Getting to Know Me Board Game and can be used daily. The book focuses on connections and relationships in the individual's reality. Information discovered through understanding an individual's life story can form parts of their person-centred care plans. The gathering of life story information, completing the book and creating care plans support and encourage family involvement.

A person's life story is never finished and the Getting to Know Me Book reflects this, as there are pages in the rear of the book where new memories can be recorded through description and photographs. Staff members can record and photograph occasions where individuals have enjoyed activities, outings and special moments. This has proven to be extremely supportive and appreciated by families who are worried, anxious and feeling guilty about having to make the very difficult decision of placing a loved one in a care home. The information recorded in the back of the Getting to Know Me Book evidences people having fun and experiencing pleasure and joy. The book is something that can be used and enjoyed by others, such as grandchildren. The Getting to Know Me Book provides families with a memento and keepsake of their loved one.

Creating a life story book can help to facilitate longer-term memory recall, emphasising what people can remember rather than what they can't. Reminiscing and sharing stories with others can enhance a person's self-esteem and improve their well-being. Only a few days ago I sat with a lady who was sitting alone at a table. I asked her if I could join her, to which she replied, 'Yes.' I introduced myself and she told me her name was Grace. She asked me what I did and I told her that I was a nurse. As we talked she told me where she grew up and that she worked in a searchlight regiment during the war. I asked her if I could write down her story in her own Getting to Know Me Book, which she agreed to. Grace laughed and chuckled as she recounted how she met her husband at a dance in Piccadilly, London. She described how he took her back to camp in Richmond Park and they kissed goodbye at the camp gates. Grace shared her memories of taking and giving messages in her war work and plotting the positions of enemy planes. Grace thanked me for talking to her and said that she had enjoyed sharing her memories with me. I then recorded them in her Getting to Know Me Book.

Every opportunity should be used to positively connect with each resident, such as during personal hygiene and being assisted during meal times. It has been during assisting a person to wash or bathe that I have found out so much about their memories, likes, dislikes and fears. When introducing the Getting to Know Me Books they were received with interest and excitement. However, there was a tendency for staff to hand over the books either to relatives or to the activity team to complete, rather than direct care staff taking ownership of the activity. The challenges that resulted from these actions were that if the books left the home they tended not to return, and, in some homes, if the activity team completed them it became a task rather than an activity that created therapeutic trusting relationships. It was important that the resident's key workers took the lead in the process of collecting the resident's life story, and in homes where this happened. the key workers' knowledge of residents' life stories was evident to see. Taking a lead facilitated the staff to connect and build relationships with the residents and their families. However, in order to increase the benefits of the book it was important that it could be used and enjoyed by others. The books were kept in a designated safe place in residents' bedrooms. Relatives were able to use or look at the book when they visited, and staff teams were able to add to the book as they discovered information about the resident.

When I talked with care workers about the importance and benefits of creating life story books for their residents, they frequently responded by saying, 'We have asked their relatives and they won't tell us anything.' On occasions, the care workers were left with the feeling that the relatives were being obstructive and unhelpful. This was generally not the situation. To remember and share memories about their relative living with dementia can be distressing for some as it reinforces just how much of their loved one has been taken by the disease. Using my experience of being a relative of someone I loved dearly who was living with dementia I explained how it can feel for relatives. I described it as like seeing your loved one put onto a small row boat and pushed out to sea. The further the boat drifts out towards the horizon the more of that person the relatives are losing. Relatives instinctively want to try to pull the row boat back to shore. They often demonstrate this by challenging the individual's memory, asking questions such as 'What did you have for breakfast?' or 'Where did you go yesterday?' One of the important roles of care teams is to enable and guide relatives to support their loved one and make their journey as calm and comfortable as possible.

In 2015 a report was published following three years of research into life story work in dementia care (Gridley *et al.* 2015). In the research findings relatives of people living in a care home believed that care staff and other professionals did not use life stories. Relatives stated that even if life stories were used by staff they did not know how often they were used.

The research also found that staff members in care homes and hospital wards viewed the making of a life story as a one-off event rather than a living document that could be added to over time. A person's life story does not end because they are in hospital or moved into a care home.

Observing relatives visiting the care home, I frequently saw visitors sitting next to their loved one often appearing lost for things to talk about. Visitors appeared to struggle to find ways to reconnect with the person living with dementia. I wanted to find a way to help people to connect – that is, between staff and relatives, staff and residents, and sometimes relatives and residents – and to bridge any gaps between these relationships.

The Getting to Know Me Board Game

I wanted to create a way of discovering someone's life story that would be fun and build therapeutic friendships and relationships. It was when I watched some residents in a care home playing a board game with laughter and bantering between them that I got the idea of creating a board game that would bring people together in a journey of discovery.

If the game was going to be played by people living with dementia it needed to have some familiarity about it that would be recognisable and was possibly still retained in the players' long-term memory. It was for those reasons that I chose to base the game on snakes and ladders.

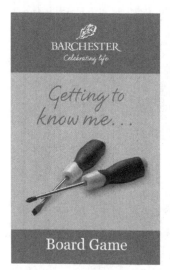
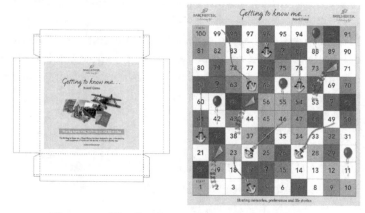

Figure 1.1 The Getting to Know Me Board Game

In this game, however, players go up kites and balloons and down the ropes and anchors. Each player takes it in turn to roll a dice and move their counters. Each player picks up a coloured card corresponding to the square on which they have landed.

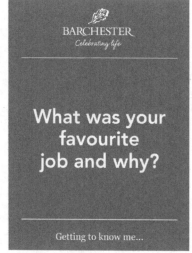

Figure 1.2 The front and back of a card

As the person plays the game and answers the questions a life story is being discovered. Each of the discoveries shared can be recorded in the Getting to Know Me Book.

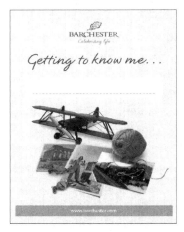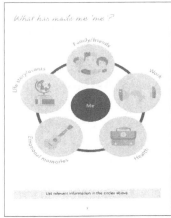

Figure 1.3 The Getting to Know Me Book

The game can be played on a one-to-one basis or as a group activity. Playing the game creates opportunities for staff and relatives to also share their own life stories.

The Getting to Know Me Board Game can be played by residents, staff and visitors together, and the Getting to Know Me Book provides something that residents, visiting relatives and friends can look through. The process of gathering and recording someone's life story information enables staff members to connect and build relationships with people living with dementia and their families.

The level of a person's involvement or participation should not be underestimated: when prompted by the right cues, people can display surprising levels of recognition. This was evidenced during games when people who were not participating in the game, but sitting close by, would answer some of the questions asked. Also, participants in the game answered questions on cards that other players had been asked. Finding time to play the game together and recording discoveries in the Getting to Know Me Book can provide individuals with a meaningful and stimulating activity.

Some people may question why the Getting to Know Me Book is being used, particularly if the person we are caring for may be unable to communicate verbally. Explaining that it creates an enjoyable opportunity to revisit old photographs and memories, and is a way of getting to know more about each other, tends to be a reassuring and acceptable response. They may be further reassured and motivated when it is explained that the book may be a beautiful gift for children or grandchildren to help families find out more about their heritage. I know from experience that we get to an age when we think, 'I wish I had asked questions when I was younger,' as unfortunately the generations before us are no longer around for us to ask. Playing the Getting to Know Me Board Game and completing the Getting to Know Me Book record the answers to those questions we wished we had asked when we had the chance.

The game can be played in five different ways:

- The game can be played using the Getting to Know Me Book.

- The game can be played on its own.

- The cards can be used on their own to initiate group or one-to-one discussions.

- The game can be played in a group.

- The game can be played on a one-to-one basis.

Outcomes of using the Getting to Know Me Book and Board Game

Caregivers' attitudes towards and knowledge of the people living with dementia and their relatives appeared to improve significantly. There was the realisation that residents had a wealth of memories and experiences prior to moving into the care home. There was the recognition that relatives had been on an emotional rollercoaster watching their loved one proceed on their journey living with dementia. This was evidenced in the writing of individuals' care plans, which became more person centred and focused on individuals' strengths and abilities. Individuals' well-being assessments improved and episodes of distress reduced.

Staff members, residents and residents' relatives made the following comments about playing the game and using the book:

It gave me an opportunity to really get to know and understand that the residents had a life before they came here.

The Getting to Know Me Book and Board Game helped in getting to know the residents' lifestyle previously and their behaviour now.

By marrying the two together we are able to recognise the residents' reality. This has significantly helped us, as a team, to move into the residents' reality and in doing so reduce their distress.

Staff are able to approach and talk to relatives more confidently.

Staff really seemed to understand Mum, and Mum seems so much more relaxed when I visit.

It enabled us to build up a rapport with residents' relatives if we had something to approach them about.

Some visitors now seem more able to speak to us when they have concerns.

From my own personal and professional experience I believe that the key to excellent person-centred dementia care is knowing the people that we are caring for. I accept that we need to recognise and understand all the different types of dementia, but we cannot cure them. However, what we can do is make the lives of those living with dementia better. It does not matter what we use to get to know someone, such as talking mats, reminiscence groups or the Getting to Know Me Book or Board Game. What does matter is what we do with all the discoveries made. We need to record them, share them and use them to connect positively with the people living with dementia, making each moment we spend with people an opportunity to make their lives better.

2

Reminiscence in the Digital Age and Its Influence

CLAIRE PEART

✳

This chapter will provide an insight into an intervention developed to offer support to residents in a care home during periods of distress. This was developed to provide stimuli for residents who initially may not respond to verbal or tactile methods of communication during periods of distress, however it may present. The chapter will look at the ways to break down the effects of the intervention to identify even further the positive engagement and activity that support the overall wellbeing of the resident.

Communication and reducing distress

Having worked for many years supporting people living with dementia in a private care environment, I have had the opportunity to spend time with some remarkable people who have helped me to develop skills to communicate and engage positively during times of happiness and enjoyment but also during times of extreme distress and ill-being.

Communication is paramount in everyday life. We communicate in so many different ways, verbal and non-verbal being the two most obvious, but we need to be mindful that people use these two forms of communication in hundreds of different ways. We need to think about different languages, dialects and accents as well as restrictions to verbal communication such as illness and disability.

We each communicate our feelings, desires and wishes differently even when using the same method of communication. We therefore need to be mindful that when we support people who are distressed we need to take a step back and process what is happening before rushing in to offer comfort and support.

It is a natural human instinct to offer protection and comfort to someone who is upset and distressed, but this is not always possible when the person is living with dementia or cognitive impairment. The person cannot always initiate contact or express emotion effectively and it is often the case that care staff need to anticipate and facilitate this. Quite often, with all the good intentions in the world, we get it wrong and inadvertently cause more distress and confusion for the person when our ultimate aim was to help.

During my time working in a care home offering support to people living with dementia who also had quite complex needs, I became involved in music therapy. This was an intervention that was supported by a qualified therapist with extensive knowledge of supporting people at various stages of their journey with dementia. The time spent with the residents was very much directed by the presentation of the resident, and Ralph, the music therapist, would 'go with the flow' and deliver the intervention at the pace the resident dictated. This did often result in quite a noisy environment, but one that demonstrated a feeling of happiness, fun and quite often euphoria.

Staff were encouraged to become involved in the group sessions that took place every Wednesday afternoon and engage with the residents, again in whatever way the residents wanted. Whether this meant singing, dancing or playing an instrument, the staff would be part of an activity that allowed and encouraged the residents to be creative and have fun. Staff would then write a reflective entry in the residents' care profiles, documenting how the activity and engagement had been positive and how they had enhanced or maintained the residents' wellbeing. The observations and information obtained were then used to develop a care plan supporting the social aspects of the residents' care, which enabled the staff to offer meaningful activity for the residents based on the interaction and engagement they observed.

Staff were initially a little reluctant to 'let their hair down', but this was short lived and the sense of wellbeing and enjoyment the staff experienced was apparent. This resulted in staff being able to connect with the residents, to step away from the 'caring for' role and become a part of the residents' social network.

In most cases, the effects on wellbeing were visible for the residents who were involved in the sessions. Residents would become animated and vocal when lyrics were recognised. Though emotions were often challenging, the bond and the connection between staff, family and residents was obvious.

Sometimes staff would need to support residents who were experiencing distress, but staff often found that by letting the resident 'find the music' as they walked around, observed and supported by a staff member, over a period of time the resident's presentation would become much more relaxed and open to conversation and communication from the supporting staff.

Historically, music has been successfully used in reminiscence-type activities and much emphasis has been placed on its benefits. 'The benefits [of the use of music] may include psychological improvement, intellectual stimulation of speech and mental processes, physical sensory stimulation and motor integration' (Aldridge *et al.* 1993, cited in Beck 1998, p.1).

The development of a new dementia care programme within the company gave me the opportunity to explore the possibility of creating an intervention aimed at everyone within the care home setting but specifically aimed at looking at ways to support our residents during times of distress. I wanted to develop something that reflected the observations made previously during the days of music therapy in the care home, allowing the resident to 'find the music'. However, I felt that something needed to be introduced which looked at more than just playing music or making sounds, and that more emphasis needed to be placed on the other ways people communicate.

Over the years there have been many projects looking at how improving the way reminiscence therapy is delivered can have a positive effect on an individual's wellbeing. Some studies have focused on older adults, responses to computer interfaces such as sharing and responding to digital images (Apted, Kay and Quigley 2006). One such study, involving the Computer Interactive Reminiscence and Conversation Aid (CIRCA) system, consists of a collection of archival media content, which is used via a touch-screen method and usually depicts images, links and videos of a city or neighbourhood where the person lives. The project lasted some time and concluded that 'during reminiscence therapy sessions, viewing the archival footage increased engagement amongst participants who normally reacted poorly to traditional reminiscence' (Gowans *et al.* 2007, p.25).

Developing a digital intervention

I initially looked at the various ways that staff in the care homes offered visual and musical stimulation and found that the main thing being offered at the time was the use of DVDs, films and so on. I felt that this was quite often used as a social intervention, frequently freeing staff up to be involved in other areas of care delivery or tasks while residents were involved in something enjoyable and interesting. If residents were showing signs of distress or preoccupation staff would often try to engage with them using various books containing pictures, information and reminiscence from previous hobbies or occupations. This was observed to be something the residents enjoyed and could often be seen to positively engage in, and it was also an activity where the staff member and resident would sit together and take part in together.

Residents face difficulty with sensory overstimulation which may increase distraction, agitation and confusion (Day, Carreon and Stump 2000), so to positively support the distress we needed to have something that could be used in an alternative environment, again reflecting on the theory of 'finding the music'. I therefore decided to produce a series of pictures from different eras (the 1950s and 1960s) and also chose different music, again from that period, to support the pictures. This was quite time consuming and, being born in the mid-1970s, it was sometimes confusing for me to positively identify what it was I was looking at. Consequently I decided to also use text in the presentations to enable staff or families to be able to positively engage verbally with the residents to encourage meaningful communication and reminiscence. The text would also help to support the resident if they were having difficulty recalling what they were seeing or listening to.

My son James works in television media as a programme editor so he assisted me in putting it all together and developing a digital show reel to play via a USB port on a TV set.

The show reel includes different topics that are accompanied by music from the same decade and changes at a rate that would allow the resident time to process what they were seeing and hearing. The topics included 1950s fashion, historical events such as the Coronation, movies that were released during that decade, and TV programmes from that period. Each show reel lasted around 20 to 25 minutes.

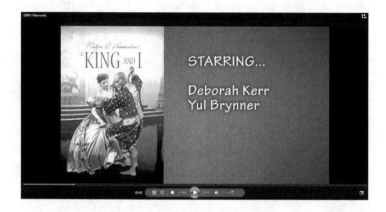

As the new dementia care programme was to be trialled in a selection of care homes throughout the UK, this served as the perfect opportunity to introduce the show reel to see if it could positively enhance wellbeing. To assist us in using the show reel to support residents during periods of distress, the decision was made to place a plasma-style TV on a wall in a corridor that would often see residents walking or gathering. We asked the staff if they could identify any corridor or area where residents had expressed some distress to see whether we could place a television in this area to see how or, indeed if, residents engaged at all with the show reel playing. Seating was also provided in these areas to support residents should they show interest in the show reel.

Staff were really keen to support the development, and felt that it may be a positive interaction, but the emphasis was made that the initial intention for using the show reel was to support staff to effectively manage distress and not as a form of reminiscence for a group of residents.

There were a few conversations held with members of the company's health and safety team to ensure the correct tests and risk assessments were carried out and to ensure that fire regulations were not compromised.

Staff were introduced to the show reel as part of the initial presentation of the dementia care programme, and the aim of the show reel was explained in some detail. Staff were encouraged to use their experiences of working in dementia care to see if they could identify people they had cared for who may have responded positively to an intervention such as the show reel. Families were also given the opportunity to ask questions about the rationale for the TVs in the corridors and, again, most of them welcomed the intervention and the possible outcomes.

As well as the use of the show reel in looking at ways to support residents during distress, as part of the new dementia care programme various clinical tools were introduced to assist the staff in supporting and enhancing wellbeing. Staff were also given training in regard to person-centred care and distress reactions, which gave them knowledge of the best ways to support residents living with dementia.

In the early part of the trial across 12 of the homes, TVs would often be turned off, and when staff were asked about this it was expressed that – more often than not – staff were not sure how to turn them on, or they felt they were too noisy, and so on. Again, the rationale would be explained.

There were a couple of times when the show reel was being played to a group of residents in a lounge as a social interaction activity and, again, although this was a positive interaction, the corridors would be left without any stimulation for those residents who for whatever reason did not want to take part in the group activity.

Staff also attended various training workshops that were developed to support the model of care used within the 10-60-06 programme and to give them the knowledge and skills to enhance and maintain the residents' wellbeing. It was during these workshops that the show reel could be further explained, in particular how staff could evaluate their observations to be more proactive in providing dementia care to our residents and in developing person-centred care plans.

As discussed earlier in the chapter, people communicate in various ways, using many of their senses and functions; during my time working in care homes, residents would often be observed by staff to use verbal communication to express needs and choices. Staff understood to some degree the importance of validation in relation to supporting a resident's reality, but quite often there appeared to be a lack of evidence that showed effective support, especially in relation to reducing distress using other, non-verbal forms of communication and for people with altered sensory issues such as residents with hearing or visual impairment.

Staff were given support to identify which different aspects of the show reel worked. Was it the visuals as opposed to the sound? Or was it the fact that the staff knew what the pictures were and thus had the confidence to fully embrace and connect with the resident during distress? Including text in the pictures made them more of a tool to enable a two-way discussion between staff and resident instead of a resident-based communication or discussion.

Again the emphasis needed to be on the person and their unique ways of communication. Staff needed to understand the positive effects of person-centred care to enable them to fully understand the way the resident would and could react to the show reel.

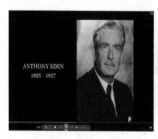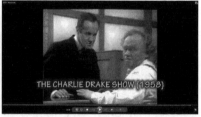

A common and central concept of understanding the sense of self of people with dementia is 'personhood', defined as being a human. Being understood to be someone unique is something that strengthens the feeling of being a human and is a prerequisite for human encounter (Kitwood 1997).

By respecting the person's uniqueness we allow that person to experience their environment by removing the barriers so often enforced on the resident in a caring role. Expression of emotion is a unique way for a person to communicate, and how that is interpreted can either enhance or devastate the person's wellbeing. As such, staff need to support the resident's freedom to explore, react and communicate however they choose, to enable a connection to be made which will allow the staff to react positively to the behaviours displayed and engage with the resident.

From observing residents as they begin to listen to the music and supporting and observing how a resident interacted with the intervention, such as dancing, singing or standing watching, the staff could understand which part of the show reel had had the most beneficial effect on the resident and could then look at ways to support this further. This understanding of the engagement and also a good knowledge of the resident's life story then enabled the staff to incorporate aspects of the show reel in effective person-centred care planning in relation to meaningful occupation and activity. This became a very proactive way of reducing episodes of distress, increasing effective communication and enhancing wellbeing.

Staff were also given a new assessment tool to help to identify triggers for distressed reactions and to work through a series of possible ways to support the residents, to ensure their needs were fully addressed and that the best possible care could be given. This tool looked at environmental, clinical and physical issues, and clear evaluation of the outcomes also ensured effective proactive care planning.

Some of the challenges we faced

Throughout the pilot of the show reel there were a number of challenges. As mentioned earlier, sometimes it was a matter of the televisions not being turned on. As the pilot continued, staff reported that some residents would become frustrated with the show reel, especially if it was situated outside their own bedrooms and was on for very long periods of time. Staff also reported that at times the footage on the show reel could be a little monotonous and residents appeared to become bored with it; they felt that more variety would be of benefit.

Staff were reminded that the aim was to reduce distress, and that they may need to look at the times that the show reel was played. If they felt that distress was heightened at certain times of the day then maybe the show reel should be on at those times only. The aim is that the resident interacts and engages, and does not become bored and frustrated by what they are seeing.

Staff were reminded that it was something that needed continuous support from themselves and not something that should be used as a form of diversion only. Their observations of the residents' reactions were key to ensuring effective use and care planning.

On reflection, and moving forward, the intervention could be something that we develop on an individual person-centred level to support people who have some history of becoming distressed: something that we develop alongside their personal life story work and incorporates the things we know are important to them. Developing an understanding of an individual's preferred choice of music is a perfect example of how having that in-depth knowledge, incorporating someone's uniqueness, is para-mount in developing person-centred interventions and meaningful occupation.

Using show reel footage of stages of the person's life with accompanying music and text is also another way for people to engage and this could be used for people who are in a room alone, such as a bedroom, during periods of distress. These could also be used on the TVs in the corridors to help other residents, family members and ancillary staff (who may not have access to care profiles), have some understanding of the person and give a clearer picture of some of the resident's life story, to possibly improve communication between themselves and that resident. As these show reels may contain personal information pertaining to the resident, consent and capacity may need to be supported.

What were the outcomes?

The show reel was piloted in 12 homes over a six-month period. Some homes used the show reel a lot and some used it a lot less, but overall the feedback from staff on its effectiveness in supporting residents who were experiencing distress was very positive.

For one gentleman who regularly became distressed, especially during and after receiving assistance with his personal care needs, music was incorporated into his care plan as a result of the staff observing how he reacted to the show reel in the 10–15 minutes following interventions. Staff then tried the approach of having similar music on in his bedroom prior to supporting him with his hygiene to see if this reduced the distress. They reported that the gentleman still became distressed but over a period of time he became much more accepting of the need for personal care as staff used the music stimulation in different ways. At first they used the show reel, then music in his room, to the point where staff would engage with him, singing and showing him pictures that had meaning for him prior to even the faintest mention of hygiene. These included pictures of his family, social interests, and so on. Staff would sing along to whatever was being played and ensured they did not cause confusion or increase distress. This took quite some time for the staff to identify and to understand, but now that they use this technique, the gentleman's distress is much less prominent and more quickly remedied.

Staff have also reported that they have observed the residents engaging with others where there would at one point have been the potential for altercation.

I had a conversation with a relative who stated that even though the 1950s show reel that played was not their dad's favourite era (he was only 62 years old), the response to and engagement in the stimuli was something they could develop and redirect to be more meaningful to him. His dad had been a DJ and would often play music from different eras but he was a huge rock fan himself. Despite the fact that he didn't necessarily become distressed, he would often appear lonely and isolated as he walked around the unit, but his son felt that since the show reel was played he was 'more alive' than he had seen him in some time. He explained that just to know this made him feel better about leaving his dad in the care home when he left. He stated it was not just that there was something for his dad to engage with but also that he felt the staff knowing how to support people living with dementia was 'apparent and comforting'.

It is again important to remember that people express distress in many different ways, and also that sometimes the show reel may not have a positive impact on residents. This is when the staff need to understand that making the conscious decision to switch off the show reel is necessary. This is also when staff need to understand the importance of validation in regard to how they respond to sadness, grief and distress.

One lady in Scotland was unable to hear the music being played on the TV but staff stated that whenever a certain still image from *The King and I* came on she would begin to clap her hands. This was a lady who was not born with a hearing impairment but had an age-related problem, so seeing the pictures of Yul Brynner and Deborah Kerr possibly took her back to the time she could hear and enjoy the film. Staff then began to sit with her and play other films of the same era and genre, and she again began to respond happily and her wellbeing obviously improved.

Damianakis *et al.* (2010) informs us that technology can be used to support and stimulate long-term memory and support social stimulation of a person with memory impairments. This was evident in the response from the lady who had hearing impairment, as it was through her long-term memory recall that she was able to enjoy a simple intervention that staff had felt was no longer beneficial to her due to a physical complaint.

One general manager stated that, 'The installation of the TV on the unit playing vintage football has proved a great success amongst some of our gentleman residents. This has stimulated memories of periods of times in their lives.' This supported evidence of an increase in the wellbeing for the residents involved.

Not all of the above examples may be seen as direct observations of the use of the show reel with people presenting with distress, but we do need a clear definition of what distress actually is. A formal definition of distress is difficult to find as dictionaries and search engines often define it differently, but I would define it as a feeling of trouble, despair, anguish, pain and sorrow. People express this in very different ways, making it impossible to class distress as one presentation or expression. Hence people need to be open-minded to the fact that with any presenting behaviour, reaction, emotion or feeling, there could be an underlying distress being experienced, and how we deal with this largely depends on the uniqueness, wishes, feelings and preferences of the individual.

Staff need to have a sense of confidence to be able to effectively support people through difficult, distressed periods, and sometimes not having the correct technique will have a bearing on the overall outcome. Having an intervention like the show reel has given the staff a common ground to develop a way to communicate effectively with residents.

To validate the effectiveness of the show reel on residents' physical aspects of wellbeing, the following quote (from the general manager of one of the care homes that piloted the trial) epitomises what we are looking to achieve. It looks holistically at how positive wellbeing can clinically improve the residents' overall health.

> *The transformation for Mary has been remarkable. She is a lady who would switch herself off from others and face the corner or stand alone in the corridor. Now she is engaged, animated and looks to be having fun. She has a real connection to the music. This in turn has led to her sleeping and eating better, and enjoying her food and the company of others.*

If this level of increased wellbeing can be even partially attributed to the interaction and interest generated by the show reel, with further development, who knows the extent to which the clinical indicators we all so passionately want to maintain for the physical wellbeing of our residents could be enhanced. It will allow staff to use this kind of interaction to support residents with non-pharmacological interventions to manage distress reactions in even more cases.

Moving forward

As reported, the feedback from staff, families and support teams was all very positive. It showed not only that digital reminiscence therapies such as the show reel worked, but also that staff had over the pilot period gained a better understanding of how supporting the residents in a more person-centred, individual way was imperative to support physiological, psychological and social aspects of wellbeing.

There was evidence from the results obtained from the introduction of the many standards incorporated in the dementia care programme, including the use of the digital show reel, that the use of anti-psychotic and hypnotic medication had dramatically reduced. The number of falls within the pilot group had also reduced, and in most cases, an increase in weight was recorded. It was evident that the implementation of the various standards had resulted in an overwhelming increase in residents' wellbeing.

One of the key things that I have observed is the impact that the development of the show reel has had on the quality of the relationships between the residents and the staff. Staff now feel that they can be creative with the residents and have fun. They understand how to observe the residents for signs of distress and now have more knowledge and skill in being proactive in the way residents are supported when experiencing distress. They understand through the support, learning and development aspects of the dementia care programme how important wellbeing is for our residents, and also understand how they play a pivotal role through continued development in ensuring this, which is the essence of effective, enhanced dementia care.

Staff could easily use this format to develop different show reels for use in the care homes, and are also exploring the possibility of personal show reels for residents who are at very late stages of their journey with dementia. It's all about having a clear understanding of the concept and vision of person-centred care and about using this philosophy in evaluating the behaviour and emotions of the residents we care for. It's also about being open and communicating effectively with the extended care team involved in the resident's care and involving the resident's family in decision making, planning and also in the delivery of this care.

How does the intervention support wellbeing?

When taking into account the wellbeing of the residents, using a digital intervention such as the show reel supports several of the seven domains of wellbeing described. By playing music and showing pictures of a specific age or era we are supporting someone's ability to grow. We are enabling them to be creative, to sing, dance and interact with others. We are also supporting residents' self-esteem by offering engagement whereby they may recognise or identify with the intervention, and be able to interact or communicate their knowledge to others, therefore ensuring meaning and a sense of purpose.

Also, very importantly, by offering such meaning and growth we are respecting the resident's individuality and recognising and accepting their identity.

Five top tips for using show reels:

- Explain to the staff why the show reels have proved to be so beneficial.

- Involve the residents and staff in developing the show reels where you can.

- Identify an area that will be appropriate for the use of the televisions.

- Ensure families are also given support to understand the advantages of using the show reel.

- Complete all required risk assessments in relation to televisions to ensure compliance with health and safety and fire regulations.

3

Namaste Care for Residents Living with Advanced Dementia

DAVID OWEN

This chapter will focus on the use of the Namaste approach in care homes and how the use of Namaste has helped to improve well-being and increased nutrition within the care home. Namaste Care involves a blend of sensory approaches and is carried out with a small group of residents in a dedicated area. The care home in which Namaste Care was trialled was particularly fortunate to work in partnership with the team at St Luke's Cheshire Hospice/The End of Life Partnership who provided invaluable training, support and resources to the home as well as final evaluations of the programme.

The Namaste Care programme was established in the United States in 2003 by social worker and dementia care specialist Joyce Simard. The name was carefully chosen from the Hindi word that means 'honouring the spirit within', to encompass and symbolise the respect for individuals who are unable to narrate to others who they are or indeed who they have become throughout their life, therefore relying on the initiative and volition of others around them to maintain their well-being and care needs (St Christopher's Hospice 2014).

The programme involves alluring and engaging individuals living with later-stage dementia through their five senses and comforting these senses by: touch through gentle foot and hand massage; smell with the use of fragrances to relax and stimulate as well as evoking memories; taste, offering delights such as ice lollies, ice creams and yoghurts to support nutrition and hydration as well as mouth care; hearing through music and natural sounds such as birdsong and water; and sight by engaging with objects that have meaning to the person (Trueland 2012).

As part of the programme to enhance dementia care, we wanted to appraise the effects of the Namaste programme on residents with advanced dementia over a six-month period. We also wanted to try to establish the influence and impact of the care programme on family, friends and the care team. In addition, the organisation also wanted to establish whether the programme could be effectively introduced into other homes within our organisation and to investigate the assumption that Namaste Care does not command additional staff or facilities or substantial cost.

The majority of dementia care home provision supports people living with dementia to spend time together irrespective of where they are on that trajectory. This can create challenges to the quality of the service provided and it can also be challenging to the quality of life and well-being of the people living with a diversity of needs due to their diagnosis and dementia experience. This can potentially lead to staff having difficulty knowing what to say or what to do if the person is unable to respond to them verbally to give a clear indication of their needs. The programme offers the residents and staff a model of care that is focused, and an opportunity to balance the different needs (Duffin 2012).

The Namaste Care approach requires a designated area away from the main communal space, envisioned to be a safe, peaceful and comforting place for people living with later-stage dementia, and requires their families and staff to uphold this approach, consistently spending two hours in the morning and two hours in the afternoon, seven days a week, away from the main community (Simard 2013).

Sometimes, people living with advancing (or later-stage) dementia in the care home are unable to narrate and initiate their needs to others and risk getting lost in the milieu. In simple terms relationships involve three things: a situation between people, a connection between them and time spent together. Connections in care homes do not always flourish where social exchange depends on the care staff or the families to initiate and maintain them. From this conclusion we could potentially end up with solitary individuals where meaning, connections and comfort are limited or even lost (Shattell, Starr and Thomas 2007). An Alzheimer's Society survey (2007) found that a care home resident typically spent only two minutes interacting with care staff or other residents over a six-hour period, not including interaction with staff during care. The majority of care staff would consider themselves to be caring and compassionate in interactions throughout the day, but unfortunately if they have low expectations of interaction and social exchange with residents living with dementia they may inadvertently increase their disability, which can then increase the care burden and the well-being of the individual living with dementia and their family (Erskine, Moursund and Trautmann 1999).

While some losses for residents living with dementia can seem overwhelming, we can still help to nourish their well-being with consideration by providing devoted friendship, connectedness and security, and, by our presence, assisting the individual living with dementia to find meaning and joy in celebrating their life and affirming who they are (Power 2014). The Namaste approach can nurture this process, giving staff and families a real opportunity to continue and develop a relationship with a person whom they deem to be a shell of their previous self.

Families protest that they do not recognise and cannot relate to what they see before them, which is almost a contradiction in terms because the person is not lost, but the relationship as they once knew it may be (Stokes 2004). The Namaste programme potentially offers family members the opportunity for a different relationship to develop, giving meaning to their time together on their visits (Chang and Johnson 2012).

For carers to consider person-centred care, they require an understanding of the surplus of material about the person for whom they are caring and, perhaps more importantly, know how to use that information to assist and enable the resident to maintain or recover well-being; the time that is spent with residents needs to have meaning and with an understanding of their abilities (Baker 2015).

The capacity for engagement can become difficult or impossible for people at the later stages of their experience, but it is never the case that any individual is entirely unable to engage with their situation. Understanding this is essential if we want the dementia workforce to move away from task-oriented care or everybody being forced into communal activity (Ballard 2016). Understanding a cognitive disabilities model suggests a way of enabling the person with dementia to engage with the world through their senses. This brings significance and meaning to time spent with individuals at a later stage of their dementia (Allen, Earhart and Blue 1992). The Namaste approach would therefore offer an opportunity to engage at a level that would create comfort and security without testing an individual's ability.

Over the past few years several programmes and interventions have been established to offer activity and engagement to people with mild to moderate dementia, so making a positive impact to their quality of life (Simard and Volicer 2010). Equivalent programmes for people with advanced dementia are not commonly well known, reinforcing an Alzheimer's Society report (2012) stating that, too often, people in the later stages are not treated with dignity, with their physical and emotional needs going unmet.

As a dementia care specialist within a large organisation I felt that the Namaste approach potentially could address what is on offer for people in our care homes at the later stage of their journey and focus on how time could be spent to benefit the needs of these individuals. It also validates and affirms the existence of an individual to the staff and family, bringing the potential to be together and therefore become emotionally attached once again. The approach also has the potential to develop and skill people up rather than them feeling awkward and unsure of how to spend time with the individual and therefore unconsciously avoiding contact.

Empathic curiosity

Our path into the world of the Namaste Care experience began with a desire to address potential disengagement of our residents in a North West care home who were living with advancing dementia. As with any new programme, communication and preparation were vital to its accomplishment. Empathic curiosity is a perspective that individuals need to consider when analysing the perceived experience of the residents with advancing dementia in the here and now. Empathic reactions communicate gratitude of what others are going through and they help to build connection, mutuality and trust. Accepting an empathic curiosity may assist the shared argument for meaningful communication whilst nurturing relationships based upon equality rather than control, minimising disability and reducing the care burden (Bruneau 1989).

To build on the stance of empathic curiosity, we began getting the team to acknowledge that the environment and their potential minimal or loss of interactions can progress to feelings of bodily isolation and emotional non-connectedness for people living with advanced dementia. In addition, if this had been compounded over days, months and years without initiative or volition, they would be unlikely to demand more interaction to relieve their isolation. It is up to those caring to reach out to the person living with advanced dementia to enable them to live rather than exist. We always need to 'go the extra mile' when working in dementia care.

Great programmes need great leaders

At the onset of the programme there was a real opportunity knocking, and sometimes it is about taking hold and grasping these with both hands. One of the greatest resources that the home and the Memory Lane Community (MLC) had was a small core group of staff who had been part of the homes establishment for a number of years. They were driven and committed to the residents but less so to the organisation, and were frustrated, mainly due to the previous management and functioning within the home that had little direction and leadership. Unfortunately this reflected badly at the time on the regulatory reports and local relationships, with numerous individuals identifying problems but offering few solutions. To say that this home at the time was under pressure was an understatement, with the staff and the environment exceptionally busy, no one person in the team being aware of their responsibility for the residents' experience, and many people receiving different responses from staff to the same repeated request, creating a chaotic and stressful day for staff and residents alike.

Leadership is about enablement and nurture, and the home had a newly appointed manager who has charisma, a forthright personality and an empathic curiosity driven by years of experience, with intuition and emotional intelligence to boot. The new manager accepted and acknowledged the issues within the home and the MLC, and with support and opportunity from the organisation has completely transformed the home. Key leadership positions within the home, such as the deputy manager and Memory Lane team leaders, were also put in place with skills, core values and beliefs that complemented the general manager's style and leadership. The Memory Lane team has the opportunity through transition and consistent leadership to bring the Namaste principles to the community for the residents with advanced dementia.

Establishing a baseline

Initial groundwork was undertaken within the MLC to establish what the lived experience in the community was like. The Quality of Interaction Schedule (QUIS) observational tool (Dean, Proudfoot and Lindesay 1993) was used initially to provide evidence to the general manager to initiate change along with a baseline to develop an action plan with our support. The general feedback reinforced that there was no real clarity to the model of care that was provided other than a team driven by tasks that were generally completed in a controlling manner, resulting in a real impact on the general well-being of the residents who at times were looking, sounding and feeling distressed. Feedback from an observation is sensitive and difficult when the culture is in need of development, and this was given initially to key leadership people within the home, including the general manager, deputy and team leaders, along with a written report. Strong emphasis on the observation and report was placed on the people who were at the later stage of the dementia journey, highlighting that they had less engagement, because people who were not at this stage were more likely to initiate and engage and decide if they wished to continue with verbal feedback or just leave. As a result these residents got more attention and interaction.

Negotiations were held with the general manager to create team 'champions' or 'ambassadors' within the MLC who would look into the life of the people at the later stages of dementia, to work alongside and provide them with support and a rationale around our plan in creating a Namaste experience; so a small home action team was established.

There were new key people in leadership roles within the team who did have good observational skills and experience, so it was thought beneficial to let the champions or ambassadors who did not have this skill be enabled in completing an observation to get a clearer understanding of the lived experience and discover what impact the observation can have on them personally. An observation can be (and proved to be) quite dramatic and cathartic as it enables observers to sense the actual lived experience and come up with their own conclusions, reflections and questioning about themselves and their colleagues. The staff were not given formal training but were briefed and asked to take notes, and then at the end of the two-hour period to journal and reflect on how they were feeling about what they had witnessed – the practices of their colleagues and generally whether the residents had an experience that they could consider positive, neutral or negative. It was felt by all parties that this was an excellent starting point.

The Memory Lane Community has potential occupancy for 32 residents so the next part of the baseline process was to establish which residents may be in the advanced (or later) stages of dementia and may benefit from the Namaste Care approach.

There has been work completed to categorise at what stage of dementia a person is at. Some of the tools and procedures that make an attempt at capturing clinical assessments are extensive and require a level of proficiency and consistency from the assessor (Kovach 1997). The Functional Behavioural

Profile (FBP) was chosen as it is intended specifically for people living with dementia to assess functioning in three specific areas: task performance, social interaction and problem solving. What the FBP commits to is identifying remaining abilities within the residents, so it is a tool that benefits goal setting and choosing therapeutic interventions that are engaging, rather than testing abilities (Baum, Edwards and Morrow-Howell 1993). At the beginning of the programme, all of the residents were assessed to see where they were 'staged' and the residents at the later stage were identified by the champions as a starting point with potential to engage them in the Namaste Programme.

Table 3.1 Residents at later stage

Later stage	Number of residents	Percentage of residents
Less than 20 on FBP	8	34% of total resident at time

An additional activity completed with the champions and home action team was to embed this process in the form of a workshop with the knowledge and understanding of what people could 'do' within sessions, and with further information brought together to support this by myself as the dementia care specialist for the home. This was very productive as it gave more knowledge and proficiency to the home action team when supervising and educating others around the reasons why some residents were more appropriate to be included within the Namaste programme. It was also supportive of their own development and credibility as a home action team. This workshop was mainly supported by the 'Capacity for Doing' tool (Perrin, May and Anderson 2008) and the residents' Pool Activity Level (Pool 2008a) to give additional rationale to the selection of residents who could potentially benefit from the programme.

The information established who was at an advanced stage and what abilities remained, but what was also significant at this point was the level of ill-being that the residents were experiencing, and this was quantified by the use of a specialist observation tool to assess well-being (Bruce 2000). Without exception all residents living in the advanced stage had their well-being compromised as indicated by this tool at the commencement of the programme. Their well-being was continually assessed on a monthly basis using this tool along with other specialist observational tools including a well-recognised pain tool and anxiety/depression tool. These tools were used monthly and findings were followed up on throughout the programme and were reviewed at the end of the programme (see Chapter 10).

Additional thoughts and support

It is well evidenced that people living with dementia are under-prescribed pain relief as compared to their elderly population counterparts. Painful conditions are uniform in both cohorts, so this emphasises that individuals living with advanced dementia are not able to explain, or complain openly, and are often prescribed anti-psychotic medication to manage their distress. Generally pain is unrecognised by nursing home staff, who believe that less than half of the people living with dementia suffer from pain when the actual figure for a care home is 80 per cent (Napp Pharmaceuticals 2014). This was greatly evident at the commencement of the programme, with little analgesia being prescribed generally on the MLC within the home. There is no evidence that depression should be any less prevalent in people who live with dementia than those who do not; in fact considering all the elements that have been described so far, there are many arguments (and much research) to suggest it could be more common. However, as with pain, observations of distress such as restlessness, sleeplessness and agitation may result in people being inappropriately prescribed anti-psychotics, so it was felt that it would also be beneficial to take a baseline measurement of the residents' medication profile.

Educating and supporting the team was essential in creating this approach. The amount of time invested by the general manager and deputy in supervision and team meetings for the team cannot be underestimated, as it provides the opportunity for support and clarity of expectations, and challenging practices in a safe and confidential forum focusing on what Namaste Care looks, sounds and feels like. It was felt that by having this process the right staff were engaged at the start who would model this care and would therefore facilitate what was expected of others once the programme was established.

Joyce Simard's books on Namaste Care (Simard 2013; Simard and Volicer 2010) have been essential as they are the definitive working guide for Namaste Care, but without doubt one opportunity that could not be missed was the chance for key people and families to listen to the guru herself. This materialised on 11th June 2015 at a 'Namaste Masterclass' organised in conjunction with the local End of Life Partnership (St Luke's Cheshire Hospice). The energy and charismatic personality of the author and creator of Namaste is mesmerising and truly inspirational. It is fair to say that it does not stop at a master class as Joyce is also accessible through her newsletter, journals and e-mail and has demonstrated that she is more than happy to support initiatives new and established, given the opportunity. These were essential opportunities available to all the staff.

Following on from the workshop, positive relationships were also formed between the home and the local End of Life Partnership (mentioned above), which was supportive in engaging with the care home in assisting with the introduction of the programme, and took a collaborative role with the education of the team and family support. All staff within the home irrespective of role and responsibility were supported to attend the in-house workshops, which were well received. With the spade work completed, all that was left to complete was the practical aspect of the room, resources and engaging the staff.

Setting up

Although this was not a purpose-built dementia home, or by any stretch of the imagination new, it did provide lots of opportunities for the Namaste programme to take place. The home had one particular room with potential to be adapted which offered plenty of peace and quiet. It was decided that six residents could be accommodated, and so the room was adapted and equipment purchased to support this activity (see Figure 3.1).

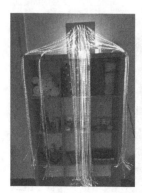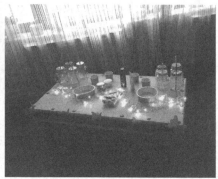

Figure 3.1 Room for Namaste Care programme

A date was set to commence the programme, and residents and their families were informed of this. Initially key staff members within the team were chosen, along with documentation and a checklist of the 'Namaste Care Activities of Daily Living' provided for each resident. It was decided that there would be an allocated time of two hours in the morning and two hours in the afternoon, seven days a week, for the programme to support six residents with advanced dementia.

The implementation and impact

The impact that the Namaste programme can have on a small group of residents living with advanced dementia cannot be underestimated. This is by no means a pampering session, but a structured process which enhances the lives of those residents who may otherwise be silent, and whose needs are often overlooked when other residents' demands take over in the general population (Stacpoole *et al.* 2015).

Once in the Namaste room, residents are individually welcomed and settled and made at ease with blankets and pillows. A selection of music or natural sounds is played and then the programme really takes shape with hand massage using aromatic creams. This gives the staff an opportunity at this point to tap into the residents' life stories using supportive objects and photographs that have meaning and significance to the individuals. This creates a mild and gentle environment where the level of stimulation can be increased or decreased with the music on the CD player along with aromas via the diffuser to give added stimulation. Another main aspect of the time is to offer nutritional drinks and smoothies. All these processes are documented by the carer on a checklist for each resident, which also includes other comfort activities such as hair brushing, warm shaves, hand holding and reading, to mention a few. This takes place for a couple of hours in the morning and then in the afternoon, with the residents joining the rest of the community outside of these times.

Namaste Care offers clinical benefits due to the more intense one-to-one contact; for example, it is easier to assess residents' pain as they are constantly within view, and it also enables more contact with massage and light movement. Assessments can therefore be completed and the residents monitored with the pain scales, and then reviewed and fed back for action to take place. The monitoring of the prescription and use of analgesia and how the residents are able to take these is also constantly reviewed and assessed, and if residents have difficulty swallowing (or reject the taste of the tablet), other alternatives are discussed and supported. Figure 3.2 supports evidence of how the programme has reduced residents' experience of pain, showing a reduction in its intensity for all residents.

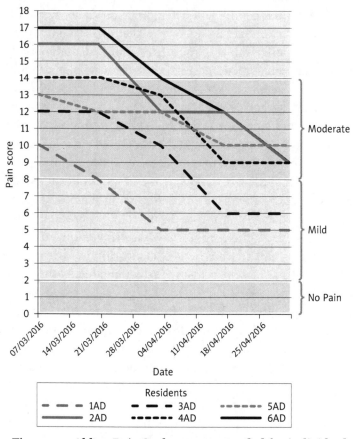

Figure 3.2 Abbey Pain Scale scores recorded for individual residents receiving Namaste Care interventions

(Reproduced with kind permission from St Luke's Cheshire Hospice (End of Life Partnership))

In a group of residents traditionally classed by some as general nursing care (rather than dementia care), and in some instances in care organisations, moving a person to a nursing unit (because it is deemed that their physical needs outweigh their psychological needs) is a common event; we considered how the Namaste approach benefits the residents clinically. For residents who were previously withdrawn with limited social interaction there were fewer periods of restlessness and intermittent infections. There were also improvements in skin integrity, and staff reported that residents were drinking more fluids which in most cases were high in calorific value, thus supporting and maintaining weight but also reducing potential urinary tract infections and added delirium. Skin integrity improvements therefore may be a consequence of increased weight and/or nutritional status while pain awareness and intense social contact also contribute to overall well-being. The peacefulness of the room and the individualised personal contact must not be underestimated in providing a comfortable and stress-free situation: when individuals had periods in the Namaste room, they were witnessed to be less distressed. This is highlighted in all residents' statistics relating to weight over a period of two months (Figure 3.3).

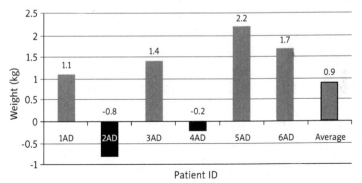

Figure 3.3 Variations in weight noted in residents participating in Namaste Care

(Reproduced with kind permission from St Luke's Cheshire Hospice (End of Life Partnership))

From the perspective of a dementia care specialist, the programme showed that distress in staff had decreased, with a positive effect on the community generally. The staff were seen with new skills, and increased staff well-being was noticeable in their demeanour and attitude; they expressed that their work was more rewarding, and had a structure that involved touch and increased interaction with their residents. This also had a knock-on effect on the relationships with residents' family and friends by helping the staff to foster closer relationships and communication with them. There was a real shift reflected in the culture of care and teamwork which had appeared to be one of 'unorganised chaos' at the beginning of the programme.

Some families before the programme began could also be described as 'lost' during the visit, and for some it was evident during observations that they appeared frustrated and distressed, attempting to reminisce and affirm who and what they were for the individuals living with advanced dementia they were visiting. Some of the relatives told us how the programme had benefited their relative and also themselves by having a more productive influence upon their relationship (and almost a rebirth). If the visits coincide with the times their relative is in the Namaste room there is now the opportunity to chat to the carer and participate in the Namaste Care experience with the person they are visiting.

How Namaste Care is incorporated into the seven domains of well-being

The Namaste approach offers time and opportunity to a group of people (living at the advanced stage of their journey) who are easily lost in the milieu of life in a care home. It is mostly visual and vocal indications of distress that are focused upon and described by staff and others. The aim with a person with dementia is not to remove the dementia, which we cannot do anyway, but to recover the person as a human being, and this is the person-centred approach that we need to bestow onto others in our care at any stage of their dementia journey.

A model of well-being is a focus to support and promote how people can live in a truly person-centred way rather than just exist (Power 2014). Namaste care provides the structure and the processes for both residents and staff to contribute in a more meaningful way throughout the day.

Power (2014) intimates that there are seven domains of well-being: identity, connectedness, security, autonomy, meaning, growth and joy.

In relationship to *identity* this is honouring the spirit of the Namaste programme. We as carers can bring and place objects of meaning and comfort in close proximity to the individuals, affirming who they are now and in the past. We must consider that the person is also a person living with their dementia and that this is part of their identity too, so that we can accept them for who they are and validate their experience and reality rather than placing them in ours. How can anybody have an identity and be themselves in somebody else's world? When a group of people live together in any setting or situation it is not unusual for the ones who can get their point across to get the most attention.

Relationships are the basis of humanity and it is the quality of these relationships that separates us from other life on the planet. One of the most difficult things to contend with in life is the loss of a significant relationship. The fact that the person living with dementia still exists in essence suggests that a relationship can still exist; what is different is that others need to adapt and adjust to have a relationship. We as carers (and others) need to accept this and cannot make people be what we want them to be. In this context this applies especially to families seeking to 'get the person back'. Until this is accepted, visits will be fraught with loss. Namaste offers time and presence and the ability to make sense without the tension of testing and wanting people back, thus providing an opportunity for all to *connect* by their presence and through the senses.

What the Namaste approach and its setting up has identified is that the people living with advanced dementia in this project, when living with the general population of the care home, constantly had distress and ill-being, but that when in a separate and engaging environment this changed, with the people feeling safe with privacy, dignity and respect in abundance through familiarity and comfort, providing a sense of *security*.

The traditional dementia community in a care home is a mix of people living at various stages of their experience. What the Namaste programme supports is a period of time seven days a week where there is a focus on the people at the advanced stage, with inclusion that is intensive and focused. We have seen that this can get lost in a dementia community with the social exchange and mutuality directed at those who can reach out to others. In this scenario *autonomy* may be lost, with an overemphasis on physical and emotional safety for the person living with advanced dementia.

The opportunity to feel needed and useful brings a sense of *meaning* to any individual. Making activities meaningful to individuals through knowing their skills and abilities supports this. We have established that meaningful activities for those at the advanced stage of dementia should be sensory and comforting, rather than testing and challenging, when using validation and reminiscence approaches or techniques. Chatting and discussing is just part of feeling needed, whereas touch, sharing and presence are selfless and mutual.

Within the Namaste programme and the room there is an opportunity to tickle all the senses, to create changing atmospheres by using the senses and creating a balance between rest and play. Examples of this include: creating restfulness via a diffuser with oils and aromas to relax, and complementing these with a fitting style and type of music; evoking times of the year and the season using smells and natural sounds; and anticipating rejoining the rest of the community through a more uplifting atmosphere rather than going straight into a more stimulating situation. The sayings 'Variety is the spice of life' and 'If you don't use it you lose it' are appropriate here. For *growth,* everyone needs opportunities to experience life in all its variety so that they can engage with the world.

Just as in Maslow's hierarchy of needs (Maslow 1954), there is a progression within the seven domains of well-being, with the first six domains supporting the seventh and final domain, *joy.* It would be almost impossible to experience happiness, pleasure, contentment, enjoyment or any form of joy without a sense of understanding an individual and without acknowledgement of that person's identity, connectedness, security, autonomy, meaning and growth.

Evaluations from others

The general manager remains enthusiastic and proud of the home for what has taken place for the people living in the advanced stages of dementia who receive the Namaste Care programme, intimating that this has enhanced teamwork, raised confidence amongst the team and fostered stronger relationships between residents, staff and relatives through its compassionate and dignified approach – an approach and culture that is now hard to break, with new team members needing to conform and fit in.

A further heart-warming outcome is that this North West home received more individual nominations than any other home within its division at the 2016 Internal Company Care Awards and is now being recognised within the local community for its dedication to its residents.

Feedback we have received from others includes the following:

We have tried the Namaste approach in one of our care homes and have observed some incredible outcomes for our residents. Staff have been really keen to participate in the programme and found working in the Namaste room really enjoyable.

[A staff member] from the End of Life Partnership gave me your contact details and said you would be happy for us to visit to see how your Namaste room works. She speaks very highly of how [the] team have integrated Namaste into what you do. It all sounds really exciting, but it is difficult to imagine it in action without seeing it and talking to staff who are doing it.

Thank you so much for showing us your Namaste set-up and taking the time out to talk to myself and [my colleague] today. We were really blown away by our visit today, the lovely friendliness of the place and the whole feel – it felt so good. It is a real credit to you and your team. So impressed with the Namaste room and how that is working; excellent feedback and results, and you can feel the passion from [the manager] and team about using the programme and the difference it makes, and more importantly you can see it from the customers experiencing it. We have come away even more excited and motivated, as we too want to make that difference. You've given us the confidence we needed to start making those steps to turn it into a reality for our customers and team of staff.

Suggested tips for others implementing Namaste Care in a care home

The Namaste Care programme did not require additional staff, a purpose-built environment or, indeed, expensive equipment for it to exist, but the deployment of the way that care is given needed considerable attention. To make it a reality there must be an acceptance and a need-to-change attitude and practice. This can only take place where there is strong leadership and teamwork. The Namaste programme will not flourish in an organisation that does not understand the philosophy that staffing has to be reorganised with care staff assigned and responsible for these residents (six in this instance), all in the advanced stage of dementia. All in-house staff must understand the philosophy and have total management backing, with a whole-home approach and cooperation from all departments, especially the kitchen, to make sure that all residents get to the venue and receive the required provisions at all times.

Education is a massive contribution to the success of Namaste Care. There still remains a mixed model of care for people living with dementia, and lots of thought needs to be given to understanding the differences between the early, mid and later stages of dementia and the impact that this has not just on the residents but the staff and families themselves. This can be completed formally in the classroom, but also with the use of qualitative and quantitative tools to continually appraise and assess. Education to support the Namaste approach also needs to involve the fact that dementia is recognised as a terminal disease. We need to find ways of preparing families to also recognise this and to see people coming into our homes as 'friends for life'.

Traditionally as the experience of dementia evolves, the individuals are no longer at risk of leaving as they are no longer ambulant. It can become increasingly difficult to engage people in occupation as they may spend lengthy periods sleeping which in turn leads to total care, and often staff seek permission to move the resident to the nursing service if the home is not secure. We must stop moving people living with dementia on to hospitals or nursing units in care homes, saying that their nursing needs now outweigh their dementia needs, which paradoxically leads to less input and increased isolation (Simard and Volicer 2010). This is a concept that as an individual and dementia care specialist I have always wrestled with internally. The expertise needed to support quality of life for people with advanced dementia at the end of their lives needs to be drawn from the field of dementia care as well as palliative care.

Namaste does not search for a reaction but uses all the senses to reach the person still inside. There may be homes that cannot create a space but all the principles of Namaste Care can still venture into everyday life in any care home. Homes can have their own unique way of resembling this approach, inspiring a fresh way to look at the palliative care needs of people with advanced dementia. All time spent with residents can be turned into a pleasurable experience rather than just being an obligation or a nursing need.

The question of difficulty in communication is often addressed from the perspective of the family or from the care team rather than from the perspective of the person living with dementia. So let us all find out who these people living with advanced dementia in our homes are, and now see the daily activity or task as an opportunity to engage with the senses – utilising touch and smell through lotions to give simple gentle hand, foot or face massages, with pleasant music and favourite tastes – in one meaningful connection. This can also support relatives and friends who find one-sided chat difficult and provide them opportunities to reconnect.

Here lies a real chance to make a difference and let people continue to live rather than just exist.

4

The Use of Doll Therapy in Dementia Care

JASON CORRIGAN-CHARLESWORTH

✳

In this chapter I will explore how the use of empathy dolls can enhance the lives of those living with dementia to promote their well-being and provide a sense of comfort. I will also discuss the best ways to introduce this within the care home environment and provide ideas on how to best support staff in its implementation.

Should we be using doll therapy in dementia care?

There are many wide-ranging therapeutic approaches adopted by care providers in the delivery of quality dementia care. The use of dolls within dementia care is one such approach that has been around for many years. Despite this fact there has been limited research into the use of this therapy, though there have been many varying views and opinions from many professionals over this period.

The use of doll therapy can be controversial and open a wide range of discussions around the appropriateness and ethical stance of such approaches for grown adults. It can also raise questions about whether the introduction of doll therapy constitutes a misleading approach by care givers and whether it infantilises the individuals provided with this therapy.

For example, Power (2014) tells us that many women living with dementia have been provided with dolls to keep or carry with them and they appear affectionate, caring and happy with them; however, he then goes on to state that a grown person carrying a doll often looks undignified or even that perhaps a deeper problem is not being addressed. Cayton (2001) suggested that enabling those with dementia to engage with dolls is a form of deceit and breach of trust, and Salari (2002) argues that old age should not be used as a second childhood, as becoming a person with dementia is not like becoming a child again.

Despite the above views, however, the Newcastle Challenging Behaviour Service were responsible for the first observational study in the UK that considered the therapeutic use of doll therapy. James, Mackenzie and Mukaetova-Ladinska (2006) looked to determine if there were any therapeutic gains to be associated with the use of doll therapy for those living with dementia. Initially, as a therapeutic intervention for people living with dementia, James et al. (2006) provided 30 toys (a mixture of 15 dolls and 15 teddy bears) to be introduced into a care home. They used a number of methods designed to help collect observational data from staff caring for the residents with dementia. The mixed-methods approach used in this study consisted of a Likert scale (a scale used to represent people's attitudes to a specific topic), which was used to measure levels of activity, agitation and happiness within the group of participants. A number of open-type questions were also used to provide a qualitative dimension to the study. It was found that in 93 per cent of the cases, residents who were given a choice of either a doll or a teddy bear preferred dolls. Also, the majority of the 14 residents who participated in this study generally appeared to be much less anxious.

Another study within the Newcastle Challenging Behaviour Service was completed by Mackenzie *et al.* (2006). The authors administered questionnaires to 46 care staff following a three-week trial providing 14 dolls for use amongst 37 residents living within two dementia care homes. Of these 46 care staff, 32 reported that the life of residents who engaged with doll therapy was 'much better', while the other 14 carers concluded that the residents were only 'a little better'. The authors, however, did not elaborate on what constituted 'a little' or 'much' better, or even whether there was an option for a participant to respond 'no better'.

While it appears that all carers believed that doll therapy had a positive effect on residents (in the form of reductions in some perceived negative reactions whilst delivering an increase in well-being), Mackenzie *et al.* (2006) highlighted several methodological issues within the study. The authors indicated that '13% of carers recorded misgivings with the study... [Some thought it was] demeaning...patronising... babyish' (p.26). It is also worth noting that 35 per cent of carers reported that there had been some problems in establishing the ownership of certain dolls, with a few arguments between residents occurring. Despite these concerns, however, all 46 care staff reported some degree of resident benefit with the use of doll therapy.

With such variation in opinions and overall findings from research to date, it therefore can still be quite confusing as to whether doll therapy is the right approach to adopt for those living with dementia. I feel, however, given the increase in the use of doll therapy within dementia care settings, that it is important to have an open mind and take a step back to look at this from a common-sense approach, being mindful that what is right for one is not always right for all.

Though I appreciate and recognise the research and views on this subject, my 27 years of experience in dementia care has put me in a position to question whether doll therapy is the right approach for everyone. I honestly feel that the answer is no, although we could quite easily come to the same conclusion about other approaches or therapies that are provided.

There is growing evidence that supports the therapeutic use of dolls for some people living with dementia which suggests that therapeutic engagement with the doll can enhance well-being, reduce episodes of distress and stimulate increased communication and social interactions (Mitchell 2016), but research also shows that we need to take a careful and considered approach to implementing doll therapy (like any other therapy or activity).

Introducing empathy dolls into care homes

As mentioned previously within the chapter, it is clear that doll therapy does have a positive impact on some individuals living with dementia, and it is with this in mind that the dementia care team decided to look at introducing the use of empathy dolls within some of its Memory Lane Communities (dementia care units) to further explore if it truly did make a positive difference to some individuals.

Whilst there are other therapies available to providers to purchase or explore, it would be fair to state that some of these interventions or activities can either be expensive, or be reliant on external organisations to provide them in the geographical area that the care home is located. In addition, some of the activities can be quite time-consuming for staff to implement. All of these factors can have an impact upon the success or implementation of such therapies, and perhaps most importantly, interaction with dolls can often be undertaken without staff members present and, from my own observations and feedback from others, will still enhance well-being.

Doll therapy in the grand scheme of things is relatively low cost and dolls are easy to obtain; however, I have never come across guidelines to assist staff in introducing doll therapy provided by suppliers of the dolls, which may be one reason why there have been some negative views on their use. One area we did discuss was the type of dolls that homes should be able to purchase, and it was felt from experience gained over many years by members within the dementia care team that empathy dolls would be best suited to use within dementia care (see the picture below).

The definition of 'empathy' according to the *Oxford English Dictionary* (English Oxford Living Dictionaries 2016) is to understand and share the feelings of another; and from previous experience, empathy dolls appear by their nature to allow those who choose to use them to show their feelings and express this via their engagement and interactions with them.

We did not want to use lifelike dolls as it was felt there may be a risk that if there was any malfunction, this could cause distress to those choosing to engage with them, for example if their eyes stopped opening.

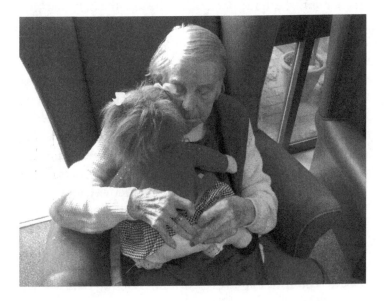

The use of doll therapy can sometimes be difficult to understand or accept for relatives of those living with dementia. However, this could be down to a lack of understanding and information provided by the staff as well as a lack of appreciation that such a therapy could bring comfort to a grown adult. I have personally never come across any other therapy or intervention that has caused such a wide range of discussion from care providers, professionals and those living with dementia as that of doll therapy. However, all would agree that every single human being has a right to be respected and have their needs met, and should be treated as a grown adult, and it could be the latter that causes such controversial debate. Power (2014) states that individuals should still be given opportunities to develop, but this may be harder to see when we position adults as children.

I would argue, however, that if a person chooses to pick up a doll and walk around with it or hold it close, this is their choice rather than the organisation treating them like a child, and it is perhaps promoting a sense of security for them. For some, if the person does believe the doll is a child or baby, by allowing them to fulfil the nurturing role, is this not promoting connectedness, a sense of identity, feelings of autonomy or growth? There are many approaches in dementia care that we may all question at some point as perhaps they conflict with our own ideas of what should or could be done, and perhaps we are basing this on our own assumptions of what we might prefer to do. For example, the same could be said about asking a person living with dementia to fill in a colouring book as an activity or complete large-piece jigsaws; is the person enjoying the activity, and if they are, who are we to question its appropriateness? To ensure we are meeting a full range of individuals' needs we need to ensure we provide a variety of therapies or interventions and therefore ensure all opportunities are afforded to people. We should focus on adapting opportunities to promote a sense of meaning.

Kitwood (1997) developed and clustered together a group of overlapping needs for individuals living with dementia: the need for comfort, attachment, inclusion, occupation and identity. Likewise, Power (2014) has asked us to consider the seven domains of well-being, as described in most of the chapters within this book and referred to within the text of this chapter. Therefore we felt that implementing a sensible approach to doll therapy will assist in addressing some of these needs for some people living with dementia within the care home whilst also alleviating elements of loneliness, distress, agitation and boredom, and providing a sense of purpose.

From experiences and discussions amongst the dementia care team we did not just want to ask the care homes to purchase empathy dolls and hope for the best. That would be both unwise and unfair for those living with dementia and also unhelpful to the staff who would be fundamental in ensuring their success. I have previously worked for organisations where dolls have just been given directly to residents or placed inside rummage boxes with no real consideration on how to best implement them or how to best observe or evaluate the impact they may have upon a person.

I have learned the hard way with a lesson that still lives with me to this day. As a care assistant back in the 1990s when I was first introduced to doll therapy in a care home, I was given a doll to use with the residents. Not knowing any differently, I approached a resident and just handed her the doll. The resident started crying and it clearly did not have the desired effect I was expecting. On discussion with her family afterwards it soon became clear that the resident in question had previously had a very sad experience during her own parenthood and this had obviously triggered some past memories. It is therefore important, as previously mentioned, that the use of such therapies requires careful consideration, and knowledge of life story events (as described in Chapter 1) is our primary focus to know if any activity, regardless of what it may be, could be suitable for an individual rather than just assuming it is.

Learning about doll therapy

Initially we devised a standard operation procedure (SOP) to guide staff not only on how to implement doll therapy but also on the importance of initially researching a person's life story, to identify (if possible) whether any such therapy may have a negative impact and would therefore require sensitivity in introducing it. The SOP also identified how to initially care-plan for those residents who could benefit from such interventions.

Such care planning must include how to best deliver doll therapy for specific residents as well as recording how doll therapy improves the individual's well-being, for example by reducing distress or anxiety or promoting a sense of purpose. Regular evaluations should demonstrate the impact that the therapy is having upon the resident in question. It is also important to note that if such therapies are seen to provide a benefit, for example in reducing anxiety, it may negate the need for certain medications (or reductions in dose) following a discussion with the person's GP.

It is equally important that staff are aware of those residents who do not benefit from doll therapy; as mentioned previously, this is not something that all residents will benefit from. This has to be recognised and understood in the same way as one would record other therapies or activities that a person may not enjoy.

The introduction of the SOP definitely benefited staff in the care homes in relation to the recording of doll therapy interventions, as it soon became apparent that there was still a lack of understanding to some extent. This lack of understanding was not just on why doll therapy may be beneficial; some staff were struggling to understanding how best to introduce the dolls and how to discuss and explain to relatives why such an intervention may be of benefit.

As a team, we then decided to evaluate how else we could further support staff working within care homes whilst empowering them to feel more confident. This was discussed in great detail, and as a team we decided we needed to develop a bespoke training/learning package to further support the implementation of doll therapy so that staff could feel more confident and knowledgeable in this area.

As with any other aspect of dementia care, best practice would be to educate those working in dementia care around specific areas that may impact upon a resident's life with dementia. We currently develop and deliver training around communication, nutrition or life story work to name but a few, so we were aware that for any specific type of intervention to be successful it requires the same level of focus and education. The development of a bespoke training/learning package in the use of dolls would allow the dementia care team to explain to relatives how doll therapy may have benefits for certain individuals living with dementia, should they have concerns or require more information in relation to this type of intervention.

Within the training session we start off by introducing staff to the empathy dolls and then go on to explain some of the many benefits they may bring to those living with dementia, including comfort, attachment, sense of purpose, security and meaning, and how they can enhance communication for some individuals. We then go on to discuss and explore how to better care-plan for the use of doll therapy, as it became apparent that more individualised details were required in addition to those contained within the SOP, including any specific style of empathy doll they prefer. We also explore if there are any particular times of day that an individual benefits from its use, whilst also stressing that doll therapy is a choice and therefore not everyone will benefit or choose to engage with it. For those who do choose to actively explain with doll therapy we also explore that doll therapy in itself is not a replacement for offering other activities or engagement opportunities, but is intended to enhance an individual's well-being.

How we introduced the empathy dolls into care homes was an important area we wanted to address so we came up with suggestions on how this could be best undertaken, for example allowing residents to show an interest first or by seeing if they choose to engage or interact with them rather than just handing them to residents and hoping that they 'work'. Allowing staff to look at residents' body language can often assist them in making a decision as to whether the doll is improving well-being or causing potential distress.

Validation approaches (Feil 2015) were another area we felt needed to be addressed, in regard to empathy dolls being referred to by those using them as a child or baby, and particularly if they used a particular name. We felt that if this was not causing distress, then best practice would be to validate the resident's reality rather than point out that it was a doll, by using a range of techniques such as asking, 'What is his/her name?' 'Do you have children?' and 'Do you enjoy it when your children come to visit?' This at first glance may appear misleading to some; however, it is no different to validating a resident who may be asking for their husband or wife or by asking if they can go to pick their children up from school: best practice would be to enter their reality and explore their feelings or to see if there is an unmet need.

It would also be important to point out at this stage that some residents may want to meet the 'needs' of their doll, particularly if they see the doll as their baby or a child they are caring for. Consideration has to be given to how the staff will address this, and respect has to be shown at all times. For example, a resident may be concerned that their doll may need to eat (and are perhaps reluctant to go for their own meal), therefore staff need to think about how this will be addressed and perhaps whether or not the doll might join them at the dining table. Alternatively, in situations like these it could be that the staff offer to take the doll for a short period to care for it.

The fantastic outcomes

Soon after introducing and rolling out the training/information session on the use of doll therapy we realised that this is what may have been missing for many years in the effectiveness and understanding of doll therapy. We feel we have empowered those who primarily provide direct care and/or activities to be more understanding and empathic in the world of doll therapy whilst making a real difference to those who benefit from its use. During the implementation of empathy dolls within our Memory Lane Communities we have also collated a number of statements and made observations, some of which I would like to share with you:

> We have one resident who gets great benefit out of the dolls. She herself was a mother to six children. She has a pram that was bought for her by her son and she uses it to push the dolls around the Memory Lane Community. It is quite clear that they bring a sense of comfort to her.

> Dorothy, who was sat in the lounge, began to look sad. A carer asked Dorothy what was wrong and Dorothy replied that she missed her husband, who had recently passed away. The carer said she was sorry to hear the news and asked if she could give Dorothy a cuddle to which Dorothy agreed. The carer asked Dorothy if there was anything she could do for her to which Dorothy replied, 'Yes, can you get me my doll from my room?' The carer immediately obliged and came back to Dorothy with her empathy doll. Dorothy sat holding her doll and started smiling and holding the doll close to her.

One man was caring for a doll which he believed was a child. He was sensitive and gentle in his dealings with the doll and was beaming with pride, showing the doll off to all around him. He interacted with the doll throughout the observation. When he became a little restless, however, he was asked if he would like someone else to look after the 'baby', to which he agreed. It was interesting to see how his belief that the doll was a child resulted in his constant attention and refusal to leave the 'baby' alone. This gentleman had previously been quite restless, walking around the community, and as soon as he was 'relieved' of his caring duties, he began to walk around again.

One lady enjoyed taking care of the empathy dolls and this was documented in her care plans, which also explained how the removal of the empathy doll would have an impact on her well-being. Staff all had a good knowledge of this and showed respect and understanding in relation to this need.

These are just a few positive outcomes that the introduction of empathy dolls has had for those who benefit from their use, although what I have been unable to capture (and is hard to explain or show you) is the sheer delight, happiness and contentment on the faces of those residents who clearly have enjoyed the introduction of empathy dolls.

Power (2014) introduces the seven domains as a way of promoting well-being and again we can see how this model could also fit in with the use of empathy dolls for some individuals.

- *Identity:* The use of empathy dolls can further promote a sense of identity, particularly if those engaging with them were themselves mothers, fathers, grandparents or even perhaps worked with children at some point in their lives, and it can also promote discussions around this.

- *Connectedness:* Those who benefit from this engagement clearly have a connection with the doll, and whether this is bringing a sense of comfort or promoting a sense of purpose, it is clear they provide a sense of engagement.

- *Security:* For some individuals the introduction of empathy dolls can provide a sense of security, promoting contentment and relaxation.

- *Autonomy:* The introduction of empathy dolls can promote elements of choice making, for example making decisions on behalf of the doll itself or using the doll to assist in one's own decision-making process.

- *Meaning:* Empathy dolls can be a way for staff to further acknowledge individuals' involvement when they are engaging directly with the doll either verbally or non-verbally, thus promoting a sense of meaning.

- *Growth:* The use of empathy dolls for some individuals can give a voice when previously they may not have engaged with others, and also allows individuals to explore and be who they want to be.

- *Joy:* Empathy dolls can promote happiness, peace and celebrations as well as improve overall well-being levels.

The use of empathy dolls can also have a huge benefit for those residents who need to be cared for in their beds and may be at risk of social isolation. The implementation of the dolls can bring a sense of companionship and love and minimise the impact of periods spent otherwise alone in their rooms. This does not imply that this is to replace the compassion, care and love provided by staff to those residents, but to enhance it.

Summary

What is quite clear from our findings is that the introduction of empathy dolls does have elements of positive impact for some people and therefore should not be disregarded even if it does not sit comfortably with others who are working alongside those receiving care. From experience, even those who initially are reluctant to implement doll therapy are quickly won over when they see the person's reaction to the doll when it is truly helping them.

As with the introduction of any intervention, in order for it to succeed we need to include, research, support, guide, monitor, record and evaluate its use on a regular basis. As somebody who has worked across the whole of the United Kingdom in different organisations, I have observed that though the use of prescribed medication to minimise distress is reducing, sadly it is still seen in some areas of the country as a first-line of approach. We owe it to everyone to explore, and where appropriate apply, non-pharmacological interventions that can potentially reduce the need for these types of medications even further.

Professor Tom Kitwood is believed to have once said, 'When you've met one person with dementia, you've met one person with dementia,' and therefore I feel that only by practising this belief and not taking a one-size-fits-all approach can we all truly deliver care that is unique to the needs of each person's rights and choices.

Suggestions and ideas for implementation

- Develop and undertake a presentation for staff on how best to implement doll therapy.

- Deliver the presentation or discuss with relatives as to why you are introducing doll therapy and address any concerns they may have.

- Explore life stories for residents to see if there may be any sensitive areas to consider prior to introducing doll therapy.

- Purchase a number of empathy dolls, including different types (give consideration to gender, race and age of doll).

- Prior to implantation discuss how you will introduce the dolls to the residents, remembering that it needs to be a choice and dolls should not just be handed out.

- Look at care planning in detail, including regular evaluation of those who benefit from empathy dolls and how they improve their well-being.

- Remember to validate the feelings of any resident who interprets the doll as something else.

- Finally, respect any resident's choice to either engage or not to engage with empathy dolls.

5

Memory Cafés

Educating and Involving Residents, Relatives and Friends

JASON CORRIGAN-CHARLESWORTH

In this chapter I will explore not only the benefits but also areas to consider when looking at developing the role of a Memory Café as part of the care home environment. I will discuss too how this resource can be used to support many people, including both those living within the care home and those living within the local community, and thus challenge the stigma around life in a care home whilst also promoting community relationships. I will also provide advice and guidance on aspects to take into consideration when looking at opening a Memory Café.

Are Memory Cafés beneficial?

In the current decade, Memory Cafés are becoming an ever-popular resource and are opening up both nationally and internationally as a way of providing advice and guidance and supporting relationship building, as well as a way of informally supporting those living with dementia and their carers. I would point out at this stage that Memory Cafés in the United Kingdom are not to be confused with memory clinics, which are formal assessment services run by the National Health Service.

The very first Memory Café was opened in 1997 in the Netherlands and was the idea of Dr Bère Miesen, a clinical old-age psychologist (Jones and Redwood 2010).

Dr Miesen chose the name 'Alzheimer's Café' rather than 'Dementia' or 'Memory' 'Café', as it was felt that most organisations for people with dementia across the world were referred to as Alzheimer's societies, even though such organisations also provide support and advice for the many other types of dementias and their related impact upon an individual. Alzheimer's disease was, and still is by far, the most common form of dementia, hence the word 'Alzheimer's' was chosen.

In his contacts with people with dementia and their families at the time, Miesen had noticed that talking about the illness, even between partners or within a family, was often taboo. Miesen stated that making dementia 'discussable' and providing information about it and its consequences were very important for the acceptance of the illness, so much so that he thought that it would be good if all those involved could meet each other in a 'relaxed forum' to exchange experiences and to talk about dementia. Dr Miesen was quoted as saying in 1999 that, 'Dementia is a complete catastrophe. Both the person with dementia and their family deserve to be well supported' (cited in Jones and Redwood 2010, p.4). Of course no one would argue with the latter point in this quote; however, the way in which individuals and their carers are supported still remains somewhat of a postcode lottery within the United Kingdom.

Brooker (2007) tells us that dementia is the most feared aspect of ageing. It is misunderstood by many. People with dementia suffer prejudice both because of their age and because of mental decline, and though there have been some improvements in this area, mentioned below, I agree that even today as a society we still come across many 'isms' that mean individuals require support and a voice to continue to fight these.

Various publications, such as the National Dementia Strategy (Department of Health (DOH) 2009), Department of Health policy on dementia (DOH 2015) and the implementation of the Dementia Action Alliance group, to name but a few, have clearly started to steer us in the right direction and have given a voice to those living with dementia and their carers, but there still is a long way to go to ensure that best practice is implemented and shared.

Background research into identifying if Memory Cafés can be beneficial has to date produced differing views due to the variation on how they are organised and run. Toms *et al.* (2015) found that two recent systematic reviews undertaken by the National Institute for Health Research on support groups for people living with dementia concluded that whilst there were subjective benefits, no conclusions could be drawn on whether they promoted positive psychosocial outcomes. This view would appear to be in line with research undertaken by the Alzheimer's Society, released in 2016, showing that 42 per cent of people mistakenly thought that once a person living with dementia stopped recognising loved ones, they didn't benefit a lot from spending time with them (Kemsley 2016). A second survey carried out at the same time found that of 300 people living with dementia, 64 per cent felt isolated from friends and family (Kemsley 2016).

Despite the above findings, research undertaken by Dr Dow (2011) into the benefits of Memory Cafés in Australia found that they promoted social inclusion, prevented isolation and improved the social and emotional well-being of the majority of those who attended. Bryden (2005) tells us that, 'We need all the support we can get, after having what I think is one of the worst diagnoses anyone can get' (p.131). Therefore one could be confused when trying to come to a concrete conclusion as to whether attending a

Memory Café does actually make a difference to those living with dementia and their relatives.

That said, I would state that it would be a fair assumption that Memory Cafés can provide support and benefit to some individuals, as with any support group, regardless of its client group, and it would depend on the exact role and remit of such environments along with the expectations of those attending as to whether they provide an overall benefit.

As mentioned previously, there are many Memory Cafés located within different towns, villages and cities all over the United Kingdom, and that popularity in itself may identify that they do actually provide a benefit. However, these Memory Cafés are predominately accessed by those still living within their own homes, and so access to them for those who live within care homes and their relatives can be very limited, as either travelling to such venues can be an issue. Additionally, as I have experienced from a personal perspective while caring for a relative living with dementia, the number of available places can unintentionally create a selection process or priority may be given to those who are perceived to be at greater risk of isolation.

Implementation and introduction of Memory Cafés within care homes

Before we explore the best ways to implement Memory Cafés within the care home environment, the reader may be wondering why I chose the expression 'Memory Café' rather than 'Alzheimer's Café'. I personally feel this makes it sound more inclusive, as the word 'Alzheimer's' could indicate that it is purely for those living with a specific form of dementia; also, there are still many individuals who have not received a formal diagnosis and the word 'Alzheimer's' may give the impression that those individuals would be excluded.

One way of enabling the benefits of Memory Cafés to become more accessible to all those living with dementia and their relatives, regardless of where they live, is for care homes to look at how they can best develop this resource and by so doing also provide a support network for relatives; this is what our organisation has looked at promoting.

It is important to point out at this stage that Memory Cafés are not intended to replace other current practices that are in place, such as residents' or relatives' meetings, or to seek their views of the care provision, as this should be covered elsewhere. The remit of the Memory Café is to build upon ways in which care homes can provide an additional resource not only to further support those they care for but also as a forum for their relatives. This can be achieved by ensuring the environment promotes and supports relationship forming, companionship, inclusiveness, understanding and fun whilst providing guidance and compassion. The Memory Café can also be a good way to explore and identify other ways of meeting current or any future needs in relation to information giving, educating and training delivery in an informal, safe and non-judgemental environment.

Within the organisation, we also believe that there is still a lot of living to do, not only after diagnosis but also after moving into a care home environment, and Memory Cafés can be another method to continue to promote and support this belief.

When I first looked at developing the role of a Memory Café within the care home environment, my first consideration was for it initially to be a resource for those living within the care home as well as their relatives. I also hoped that a Memory Café within a care home could broaden its audience by opening its doors to those living with dementia and their carers in the area. I envisaged the ultimate role of the Memory Café as being beneficial in some way to all those who attended, including relatives and carers. I did not want it to be seen as a place to drop off a loved one, but a way to enjoy activities and spend time together whilst enjoying the company of those with common interests and common experiences. It was also my intention to provide a resource where information and relevant training could be provided when required to further support all those who attended, and a way of further enhancing community links.

I thought that by developing this opportunity, it could also be a way to promote the positive role of care homes within their localities and to be seen as a hub of support and guidance to all those living with dementia, whilst disproving some of the articles in the press that suggested that care homes are not always a good place to live. For many people living with dementia in the community the reality is that eventually a move into a care home is inevitable and therefore promoting those relationships and showing all the good work care homes actually do could make the eventual transition somewhat less stressful and provide reassurances to all those involved when that time came.

I was very mindful that exploring this overall specific remit of a Memory Café would involve careful consideration as I did not want to cause distress or impede on those who actually live within the care home. Ensuring there was adequate space to run such a resource was crucial whilst respecting that some people may choose not to attend and that these individuals should not be asked to change their routine to accommodate a Memory Café. That said, however, I do believe that care homes have a place in promoting community links and feel this was an excellent method to do so. After all, in 2012 the Prime Minister, in partnership with the Department of Health, published the *Prime Minister's Challenge on Dementia* (DOH 2012), part of which discusses the need for more dementia-friendly communities. Promoting the role of Memory Cafés particularly within care homes can, I believe, be one way of assisting in promoting this value.

Articles written around the roles of Memory Cafés have variations in their remit for such environments; however, I wanted to develop a fluid setting that had variation in what it provided (as previously mentioned), thus ensuring it was reaching out to everyone who may choose to attend. The first avenue to explore was in relation to the environment (given that care homes vary in size and communal spaces available); this was an area that required careful consideration.

The care home where we initially looked at setting up a Memory Café had the benefit of a separate communal area and therefore could be utilised without impeding on the running of the home or those who lived there who may have chosen not to attend.

Given that we wanted to look at a Memory Café that was going to be accessed by both those living in the home and their relatives, as well as those within the community, the planning and discussion had to consider all of the following areas:

- identifying key people (and their specific roles) who worked in the home who were willing to be involved in facilitating a Memory Café

- the role of relatives and carers when in attendance

- adequate parking facilities

- access by public transportation whenever possible

- accessibility for people who required wheelchairs

- adequate toilet facilities that could also be accessed by people with disabilities

- safe and easily accessible fire escape facilities

- comfortable seating and tables

- provision of a first aid kit

- provision of a selection of drinks and snacks

- a selection of games that could be used for sessions, plus the ability to play music and show films

- developing a resource list and resource library of local and national support services, should those attending require these

- identifying possible professionals/organisations that would be willing to attend to facilitate discussions, should those attending choose to learn more about dementia or specific elements of it

- possibly looking at recruiting volunteers who may wish to assist

- consideration to monitoring the numbers that may wish to attend, and exploring registration of an interest among potential attendees, as over-attendance could be an area of concern

- marketing plans and advertising the Memory Café initially for those living in the care home and then more broadly in the local community.

Once we had explored all of the above, we invited those living at the home and their relatives to a meeting to explore with them what they would like to see from the Memory Café and to share the ideas we had initially come up with. At the meeting, it became apparent that those in attendance were very welcoming and supportive of the idea of a Memory Café being set up at the home. They felt this would be a great opportunity for promoting relationships, sharing experiences and spending fun and quality time together.

What also quickly became apparent was that many relatives in attendance felt they did not know much about their relatives' condition and were unaware of many aspects of best practice in dementia care, for example, that different types of dementia have different traits or how legislation like the Mental Capacity Act supported those living with a dementia. Many relatives also wanted to know how they could further support staff when they visited, in relation to what to say to their loved one when their reality was different or why areas like life story work were so important.

Following the first meeting, it became clear that my initial thoughts on providing a fluid approach in the role of the Memory Café were accurate. It was clear that the remit of the Café would need to be dual-faceted: some sessions would need to be structured to deliver relevant information and guidance to those who felt they required it, whilst other sessions needed to be more informal and geared around fun and meaningful discussions together as a group.

The meeting also highlighted that all sessions, regardless of their content, would need clear and careful consideration about what information was delivered to those who attended. I am not implying here that those living with dementia should be excluded from potentially sensitive sessions, but that there needed to be recognition that some individuals may not wish to discuss or explore certain topics where others may be willing to; an individualised approach would need to be taken and, where necessary, best-interest decisions made. Also acknowledgement was given that some sessions, depending upon their remit, may not suit all individual needs and therefore individuals needed to be able to choose what sessions to attend or not according to their own beliefs, choices and preferences.

Frequency and times were also discussed and it was agreed by the group initially that the Memory Café should be run every second month, and also run at different times of the day including early evenings, so that it was accessible to all who may want to attend, and also that it would be no longer than two hours in duration.

Finally at this initial meeting I discussed my vision about eventually opening the Café up to members of the local community living with dementia and their carers.

The group felt that such a resource was greatly needed and would have been a great benefit to some of them as individuals earlier on in their journey, and would have provided a great support network for them.

Concerns were voiced, however, about the numbers of people the Café may attract, so we did discuss a system whereby people would have to contact the home to confirm attendance prior to attending rather than just arriving, as this could have a major impact upon the size of the room and facilities available.

One area that I did not initially envisage any concerns with, however, was that of staff confidence in taking a lead in running such sessions. On discussing the role of the Memory Café with the staff group at the home, although they were all supportive of the idea and felt confident in running various meaningful activities, they felt that facilitating other aspects of the Café would be challenging as this was a completely new concept to them, and for some it took them out of their comfort zone.

Within our organisation, we do have a small dedicated dementia team that supports all of its care homes. However, I did not want the Memory Cafés to be purely run by us as a team but to work in partnership with care homes and support dedicated sessions where more specialist information was to be provided. Realistically, it would be extremely difficult for us to be at each session, particularly if we were going to look at rolling the idea out to more homes across the business. I also wanted to empower the homes to take the lead in running these Cafés as staff would have already built up trusting and empathic relationships with the residents and relatives they already supported. I also felt that those who attended would find this approach less stressful and that they were more likely to attend if there were familiar faces present.

Moving forward

At the time of writing this chapter, the home where we were looking at developing this initial concept has run its very first Memory Café session, which has been successful; both residents and relatives who attended found it beneficial and enjoyable and this resource will continue to be provided so we can ensure we are truly supporting and providing a holistic approach to care for both those who live in the care home and their relatives.

Another home within the organisation has developed a Memory Café, but this is run by a local support group and is open to both the community and residents alike. Though this is excellent, unfortunately not all homes have such groups available to them and therefore we wanted to look at other opportunities to ensure this resource was available to all.

With this vision in mind, as an organisation we are currently working on developing guidelines for all our care homes that provide dementia care for setting up a Memory Café. This will include areas for consideration that both management and staff will need take into account when looking at developing Memory Cafés, including examples of good practice. These will incorporate how to best run/facilitate such groups from their initial setting up, to advertising such a facility, to planning a structured yet flexible programme and also how to work alongside carers and relatives to ensure that it is an inclusive setting.

We are also exploring the introduction of some kind of evaluation format that can be completed periodically for all those who are attending to ensure that current and future needs can be considered, and to allow homes to continue to develop and discuss the contents of the Memory Café format to meet any change in need or expectation of the group who attend.

One way we are also considering to support the development and success of the Memory Cafés is to align the objectives of the Cafés to the seven domains of well-being introduced by Power (2014). Each of these domains could support sessions by ensuring that all those who attend acknowledge the domain, and would give the format some clear aims and objectives. Each of these domains would fit well and, as an example, could look something like this:

- *Identity:* All those who attend each session regardless of its contents are to be included, encouraged and supported in conversations that revolve around them as unique individuals.

- *Connectedness:* Those who facilitate and attend each session ensure they are known by everyone by way of initial informal introductions and sharing similarities, and promote meaningful experiences including joint interactions and discussions.

- *Security:* A safe non-judgemental environment is provided where everyone is respected for who they are and any anxieties are acknowledged and supported. If people have moments of uncertainty then this is recognised and supported, and reassurance provided.

- *Autonomy:* Independence, choice and respect are constantly provided and promoted and any involvement, regardless of what it is, is recognised.

- *Meaning:* All contributions are recognised, supported and valued even if they differ from our own.

- *Growth:* Different opportunities are provided that promote a sense of pride and achievement, along with provisions not only to support existing skills but also to learn new ones.

- *Joy:* Supporting fun and celebrating achievements and successes.

Summary

What is quite clear from the literature and from looking at the role of Memory Cafés is that they can be an excellent opportunity to provide further support to both those living with dementia and their relatives.

Additionally, they also an excellent resource for promoting relationships whilst providing meaningful engagement and activities, and also for identifying and delivering guidance and information to an audience that otherwise may not have access to such support.

Developing and delivering such a resource clearly requires careful thought, consideration and preparation, both initially and ongoing. I truly believe, however, that by supporting care homes to look at this approach we are one more step forward in ensuring that, regardless of where someone may be on their journey with dementia and regardless of where they may be residing, everyone has an opportunity to continue to learn and to live life to the fullest potential.

Suggestions and ideas for implementation

- Look at the suitability of the environment and when choosing a space ensure it does not impede on the residents' home.

- Discuss with those living at the home as well as their relatives the purpose of the Memory Café and what they would like such a resource to provide for them.

- Develop in-depth best-practice guidelines to provide ideas and suggestions for developing Memory Lane Cafés, incorporating all areas.

- Identify key staff who feel confident and supported in delivering such a resource.

- Look at what services, whether internal or external, can provide information and give support.

- Ensure there are adequate resources to promote meaningful activities.

- Regularly seek the views and opinions of those attending to ensure it is continuing to meet all needs.

6

Linking Exercise and Wellbeing for People Living with Dementia

PHIL HARPER

❋

This chapter was written to identify various opportunities for physical exercise that are available to our residents living in Memory Lane Communities (MLC), which provide care for residents living with dementia. Utilising an observational tool, I observed several sessions of physical exercise within the care homes to establish how, whilst improving physical health, the exercise might influence psychological wellbeing. This chapter shares with you some observations of individual and group resident wellbeing levels being enhanced through the activities which I was able to observe.

Whilst supporting three homes on the dementia care programme, I spent time observing different aspects of physical exercise for residents living within the MLC, the exercise being either self-directed or more formally included in activity sessions. The main question that ran through my mind at the time was 'Do movement and exercise offer more than is suggested in prevention, maintenance and improvement of an individual's physical health?', as I recalled many occasions when I saw residents enjoying themselves during periods of engagement through exercise sessions. I therefore wanted to use my observations to highlight that the wellbeing of residents living in a dementia care unit may also be improved with the introduction of physical exercise.

So what do we mean by exercise?

The Free Dictionary (2017) tells us that exercise is 'physical activity that is planned, structured and repetitive for the purpose of conditioning any part of the body. Exercise is used to improve health, maintain fitness and is important as a means of physical rehabilitation.' In recent years there has been much research and many government-led initiatives which have put a real emphasis on physical activity and its benefits for the health of the nation. In general it has been accepted that every person has a responsibility to improve their personal health and wellbeing for a healthy lifestyle in later life, and that this should be extended to residents living in care homes.

Many people have taken on the challenge of improving their general physical health through exercise, such as physical fitness regimes provided by programmes introduced in health and fitness clubs. There also appears to have been a rise in personally driven, enjoyable physical activities, including cycling, swimming, jogging, walking and the use of exercise equipment which may be used in the home.

The fitness drive has particularly been encouraged in older age, not just for the physical benefits a person may receive but also because it has been suggested that it will reduce the risk of developing dementia. Some GP practices now 'prescribe' a series of fitness sessions at local fitness centres, allowing an older person to attend for free.

Some social groups also give their members the opportunity for physical activities, such as indoor and outdoor bowling, dancing, exercise classes and hiking.

There are even holiday organisations for the over-sixties which provide activity holidays that can be enjoyed by this age group. Perhaps the main directive for increased physical exercise in older age is to maintain good physical health whilst attempting to provide a longevity that is rich with social involvement and, for some individuals, to appear and feel younger than their age.

To assist in achieving improvement in the physical health of the older population there have been many articles and other sources of information suggesting activities that will complement the physical exercise approach to a healthy lifestyle.

The National Institute on Aging (2016) in their programme 'Go4Life' have identified four types of exercise. They suggest that exercise and physical activity fall into four basic categories: endurance, strength, balance and flexibility. Most people tend to focus on one activity or type of exercise and think they're doing enough; however, each type is different. Combining them will give an individual more benefits, and alternating them also helps to reduce boredom and the risk of injury.

Education and sharing information with the general public provides a responsible and acceptable method of motivating and encouraging everyone to be more responsible for their health needs. The *British Medical Journal (BMJ)* (2014) also provides a platform for supporting health education, and delivers learning modules for education, such as the *BMJ* learning module for health benefits of physical activity, which recognises:

- how physical activity can help to prevent depression and anxiety

- how physical activity is an important part of management for patients with depression and anxiety

- how physical activity can improve sleep and sleep apnoea

- how physical activity can reduce cognitive decline and prevent dementia

- how to recommend physical activity to patients with mental health problems and dementia.

Physical exercise and cognition

The information above links to the recent recognition that there should be consideration of the types of physical exercise and activity which may have an impact on the reduction of cognitive decline. There are health agencies and reports which now incorporate this recent thinking. Given the opinions that physical exercise can have an impact on dementia, there needs to be some consideration of research outcomes and also guidance and advice around exercise which may be suitable for people who already have cognitive decline. The physical exercises do not have to be different to the types of physical activity discussed above to enhance the health of the older person.

Do the recommended four types of exercise for the older person as suggested in the Go4Life programme require any particular consideration when introduced into physical exercise for people who live with dementia? A recent research study highlighted by McArdle (2016) regarding physical activity in dementia patients is that of van Alphen *et al.* (2016), who reported that dementia groups are more likely to engage in low-intensity activities such as walking or household chores rather than high-intensity activities which would be available for the general older population. These activities are beneficial for cardio-respiratory capacity and body composition, and exercise interventions could be tailored to suit this preference. The effects of vigorous exercise (such as sprinting or spinning) and low-intensity activities should also be compared. This is an area ripe for investigation which may be beneficial for the development of physical interventions.

With the recognition of the importance of physical exercise for a healthy lifestyle in older people, and of education, advice and support, directives are now available for exercise in dementia. The Alzheimer's Society (2014) have produced the Staying Involved and Active programme which not only relates to benefits of activity for the person living with dementia but also acknowledges the benefits that activity offers to carers, family and friends.

Physical exercise to enjoy?

Physical exercise may be represented in various forms, and my personal experience is that it needs to provide me with some enjoyment. I would rather spend an hour walking with my dogs around Cannock Chase than be sat on an exercise bike in a gym or, worse still, have a workout in my garage! This is also true for some people regarding their life journey. It's a journey that should be enjoyable. Of course for some, physical exercise may never feature on their 'wish list' of things to do but we still have a responsibility to try to encourage the residents and perhaps try to make it fun to do.

Observations of wellbeing

The observations in each care setting were carried out using the Barchester CAREFUL observational tool to identify specific outcomes for individual residents along with a general observation for all residents present in the community. The Barchester CAREFUL observational tool was designed to identify the psychological experience of individual residents living with dementia in Memory Lane Communities. It enables us to record and reflect upon the (perceived experience of) wellbeing levels which may be identified in residents who become involved in activities and interactions that the environment offers. The outcomes of this are used to identify the residents' care needs and support the care planning process.

I concentrated on the residents' wellbeing by reflecting on the seven domains of wellbeing (Power 2014). I observed physical exercises at the individual homes and will share my observations and thoughts relating to the physical exercise and outcomes within each home.

Observations from Care Home 1

I have visited the first home periodically for one year, where my presence was required in the Memory Lane Community. The home is very spacious and has quite long corridors, enabling residents to walk around the building. There have been rest stops developed to provide the opportunity for a resident to retire from walking and spend time doing as the stops suggest: 'rest'. The desire to walk may soon return and the resident continues on their journey. There may be an opportunity to have sociable interaction along the way should someone have time to stop and have a chat. What a good way to reduce boredom, and a nice way to have social interaction and to get some physical exercise to help maintain physical health and mobility.

This home also has a lovely garden with winding footpaths around the building. The garden has flower borders and shrubs, chairs and rest stops too, along with a designed themed area which represents the seaside. Doors from the lounge areas offer the opportunity for a walk not only around the garden but also from one area of the community to another. Usually, more so when the weather is good, residents are able to walk around the garden and obtain fresh air, sensory stimulation and also good physical exercise.

The rest stops in these areas were developed as part of the 10-60-06 dementia care programme, not only to provide an important opportunity for resting but also to provide a social interactive experience with other people who may also share the ability to maintain their physical activity.

With the introduction of the programme, there was also an opportunity for two staff to receive training in chair exercises and chair activities, with a focus on making these activities fun, which would be included in the group activity planner within Memory Lane. I was able to observe the delivery of the chair exercises during a 'CAREFUL' observation where a group of eight residents were supported to engage in the physical exercise along to music. I observed four of the residents during a 30-minute session.

When commencing the observation, three of the residents were recorded as having the same baseline wellbeing score, which suggested that they appeared happy, smiling, involved and thoughtful. Another resident, Stanley, also was recorded as having the same baseline wellbeing score, as he was chatting with other residents and asking staff questions regarding what was to take place. (All names have been changed to protect the residents' identity within these observational recordings.)

On this occasion a short period of warming-up exercise took place for a few minutes which allowed staff to encourage and engage with residents whilst preparing them for what was to take place. Once the music had begun residents were given the opportunity to interact with activity equipment such as balls and pom-poms, and encouraged to raise their arms up and down along with shaking the pom-poms. They would then sway their arms from side to side to the rhythm of the music. Staff also included leg exercise by suggesting that they raise alternate legs up and down. Two of the residents who I was observing, Jack and Mary, also started to rock their heads from side to side as a natural response to the music.

Jack and Mary sat next to each other and as soon as the music and exercise commenced they quickly engaged and followed the delivered programme with much enthusiasm.

Within the first five minutes of the observation they had achieved a higher wellbeing score. This score suggests that both Jack and Mary had a high level of involvement with a very happy mood. In fact they both kept looking at each other, and commented and laughed together. This continued throughout the exercise with both Jack and Mary maintaining a higher wellbeing score following the completed chair exercise, as they held onto their pom-poms during the ten-minute observation, which continued after the session had finished.

Stanley, who had initially been quite chatty and engaged with the other residents and staff, did not physically join in the activity even though staff encouraged him to throughout the session. Stanley chose to sit and observe whilst occasionally talking to residents either side of him or making conversation with the staff. During these short episodes of conversation, Stanley also managed to achieve a higher wellbeing score. These were times when Stanley was noted to have a high level of involvement and smiled at staff who were communicating with him. These episodes were not maintained, however, as in between each intervention with staff, his wellbeing score dropped. Since Stanley did not engage with the exercise, there was no direct benefit from the physical activity, because he chose to observe rather than participate throughout the session.

The fourth resident, Tom, required an activity support person to encourage engagement throughout the session, leading to a gradual increase of his wellbeing level, which took much longer to achieve than for Jack and Mary who were quickly engaged in the exercise. The activity support person recognised that Tom had difficulty following the instructions and the chair exercise. The activity support person held Tom's hands and also supported the balls and pom-poms that Tom had been offered. It wasn't that Tom did not wish to hold them but rather that Tom's dexterity and grip was reduced. The activity support person held the equipment in her hands whilst also holding Tom's hand. With some encouragement and support, Tom began to engage more and during the final 15 minutes of the programme he smiled and responded to the activity support person. It was noted that when his wellbeing score increased, the activity support person only had to support Tom's hands with one finger, whilst at the same time Tom was gently waving his arms from side to side.

The staff who were responsible for the chair music and movement exercise considered that it had been beneficial for the residents in short 30-minute sessions on a regular basis, but they also felt that there were signs of residents quickly tiring when it was delivered for longer periods. On this occasion there were certainly three residents who showed determination and enjoyment with their involvement in the chair exercises and engagement with the music.

Observations from Care Home 2

The second home which I supported for the dementia care pilot programme was a residential-care Memory Lane Community which was situated in beautiful surroundings in a rural setting in Shropshire. The availability of gardens that opened onto the views gave residents the chance to walk outside and engage with the vista, along with regular outdoor events which were very popular at this home. General physical exercise was promoted with frequent excursions on local activities such as boat trips on the canal and visits to local historic places, which promoted their physical and psychological wellbeing.

A similar chair exercise programme was observed at the second home. This was provided by an outside organisation and presented by a very cheerful and understanding lady. I completed an observation which concentrated on four residents whilst also observing a general response for all residents who had joined the activity, which was being held in the communal lounge.

Once more the session began with a warm-up by encouraging gentle exercise, inviting residents to massage their hands and stretch their fingers and hands whilst also gradually moving their arms and legs up and down. In addition, soft sponge balls were offered to residents to squeeze in their hands. The warm-up session lasted for around five minutes. When commencing the more engaging exercise, the presenter asked the residents for requests for songs and music which they would choose throughout the session; she then delivered the exercises to the rhythm of the music which encouraged a party atmosphere. The equipment included balls, pom-poms, scarves and batons which were alternately presented to individuals. Most residents joined in spontaneously, although some required further support.

The four residents whom I observed had differing levels of physical ability, along with different levels of engagement and concentration.

One lady, Clare, was 'in it to win it'; her first five minutes were recorded as being 'happy' and she listened quite intently. There then followed a surge of engagement where she was suggesting various songs and music whilst following all of the exercise routines. There were many observations of Clare engaging with other residents by vocalising and encouraging others to keep up the pace. Clare maintained her enjoyment throughout, which was evidenced by her smiles and laughter whilst extremely involved and engaged. It was only during the last ten minutes that Clare began to gradually show signs of withdrawing from the exercise programme and sat back with a more relaxed composure whilst periodically joining in with the song being played. This did, however, also coincide with the cooling-down exercises which were being delivered to everyone.

One male resident, Cyril, experienced much the same enjoyment from the beginning to the end of the programme.

He was very keen to engage with the exercise and also offered suggestions for the songs and music that could be played. Cyril was able to retain his happy and engaged mode throughout the 75-minute session with just one short period of rest ten minutes before the session ended; this also corresponded with the slowing-down and cooling-down time when the presenter was encouraging residents to be more restful.

Two female residents who required support and encouragement received intermittent care-staff involvement. One of these residents, Jane, was already engaging with an empathy doll at the beginning of the observation and this was maintained throughout the session. It did, however, appear important for Jane to concentrate upon her doll, and Jane only joined in with the exercise when staff encouraged her. However, her wellbeing levels scored higher when she joined the activity and she would instantly start to laugh and move her body, arms and feet to the rhythm of the music. Jane was able to maintain her wellbeing levels by caring for the doll whilst the activity was taking place.

The fourth resident, Susie, had a slower pace of involvement with the music and exercise. The observation recorded a neutral level of wellbeing. There were periods of increased wellbeing when Susie attempted to engage. Mainly, Susie sat observing other residents with occasional attempts to move her arms and hands and join in the singing. The session appeared to be outpacing Susie's ability to fully engage although her wellbeing levels did increase as she began to offer smiles in response to the presenter when she approached her. There was a change, however, when the activity coordinator moved to sit beside Susie and identified a need for support. With some encouragement Susie became more engaged with the equipment being used; use of the ball and the scarf, and her arm and leg movements, became more obvious and spontaneous to the music. At one point the engagement with the baton provided an opportunity to conduct the music! This supplied 45 minutes of evidence where Susie was observed to have a high level of wellbeing as a response to the music and exercise along with interaction with the staff member. Susie showed much happiness and would turn and look at the activity coordinator with a smile.

Whilst the exercise was obviously enjoyed by the residents, the staff continually attempted to maintain the residents' wellbeing by encouraging them to get up and dance. At this point other care staff came into the lounge, joined in the group and invited residents to accompany them in a dance, for which some residents showed enjoyment by taking up the opportunity.

It was during one support visit to this home that I also had the chance to complete an observation during a session of 'Bocha', which was part of an activity afternoon. This comprised a seated game of bowls where eight residents had the benefit of playing this game for an hour. It was organised by a young woman from an external organisation who supported activity for residents living with dementia.

I once more selected four residents to observe whilst also delivering a general observation of other residents during this activity session.

Residents were sat in a line at one end of the room, and the floor in front of them offered the pitch whereby one person would throw or bowl a small ball in front of them. All of those seated took turns in then attempting to throw or bowl their ball to get as close as they could to the smaller ball. The room was a quiet setting and unlike the previous observed exercises, there was no music involved.

At the beginning of the observation the residents did appear to be throwing the ball but it became very noticeable that as the game progressed the throwing action was less obvious and the bowling action became more evident. The bowling action possibly became more obvious as the game became more competitive, and the competition element was equally noticeable for both male and female players.

It was interesting to see that as the game became more engaging for the residents their exercise was more intense as they began to lean down to get their hand closer to the ground which enabled them to bowl more than throw. The bending increased their movement and the exercise was therefore more intense. It was also interesting to note that the residents' concentration and interaction was increasing and they were becoming more motivated to win. Even the occasional personal comment was used in a humorous manner!

The recording of the observation for the four residents identified that for the first ten minutes whilst warming up, the hand and finger exercise was accompanied by some conversation which was mainly such comments as 'I don't know how to play this' and 'I won't be able to do this.' All comments were responded to with much reassurance and encouragement. The therapist used some reflective discussion, suggesting that one resident was excellent last time he had played, and for another lady, 'You said how much you enjoyed playing this last week.'

Once the game had commenced, the wellbeing levels for three residents, two men and one woman, increased significantly, identifying that they were very happily engaging and involving themselves in a game in which they could interact and compete with their fellow residents. Some instruction and confidence-boosting from the therapist no doubt supported the positive response from the residents.

One woman took a little longer to become more actively engaged although she was playing the game. This was possibly due to the fact that she was waiting for a visit from her husband. After a period of 20 minutes her husband arrived and sat beside her. This further encouragement led to her wellbeing increasing as she too began to laugh and smile whilst managing to play the game as well as everyone else. At one point she did sit back and disengage from the game as she said she felt tired, and she rested for a few minutes. Her wellbeing level did reduce although she still managed to stay awake and watch the game whilst chatting to her husband. After the short rest, the woman was able to resume the activity with as much involvement as before. Once completed, the game was followed up with cooling-down exercises.

Observations from Care Home 3

The third home which I supported as part of the dementia care programme was also in Shropshire but was situated in a more built-up area near the town; their Memory Lane Community supported residents requiring nursing care. The environment provided corridors which encircled the courtyard garden, and many residents in this community enjoyed walking around the corridors which also provided rest stops and a view out onto the garden space. The garden was accessible from the corridor and lounge area.

There is a significantly higher proportion of residents who are independently more mobile in this home than in the first home I discussed, and the residents therefore provide themselves with regular exercise in the form of having a walk around the building and garden.

My visit here allowed me to make a general observation of the exercise programme I had experienced in the second home, which was provided by an outside company. This woman presented the exercise session in much the same format, providing selected music and equipment including balls, pom-poms, scarves and batons, although delivered to a smaller group of residents. One male resident, Fred, quickly engaged with the music and sang out to 'Red Roses for a Blue Lady' and other songs such as 'Spanish Eyes'. All residents in the small group (six residents, one carer and one relative) showed enjoyment and engagement with the exercise and music. One resident, Julia, danced around the room to the rhythm of the music and was totally engrossed with the experience she had been offered. Julia demonstrated her love of dancing, even without a partner, swaying and swivelling around, rocking her body and swinging her arms, loving every minute. Julia does at times become distressed but the staff identify her love of dancing and try to reduce her distress whilst attempting to increase her wellbeing levels with the use of music and dance.

Later on in the day I was also able to complete an observation at this home whilst a less formalised exercise activity took place. I recognised that the activity coordinator offers a physical exercise activity for residents whenever the opportunity arises. The activity coordinator entered the communal conservatory bouncing a plastic football whilst asking residents who wanted to join in the activity. Three men accepted the invite and they joined together in the conservatory. The warming up progressed gently, passing the ball to one another either by throwing or kicking. It appeared that the residents did not require much instruction at this level, maybe because it was an activity they regularly enjoyed or maybe because it reminded them of a football warm-up session. The football game continued with bouncing the ball as well as throwing the ball to one another. The exercise then went on to include dumbbell-shaped equipment which had a similar purpose to castanets as they had beans inside which would rattle when they were moved around. This exercise was used to encourage the residents to raise their shoulders and arms, and also to encourage arm stretches whilst calling out a beat to the count of ten. The pace of one resident, Sid, appeared to be affected by not being fully able to understand the instructions. The activity coordinator recognised the need to offer more support to him and moved nearer. He then faced Sid, which allowed him to copy the movement and this non-verbal action changed the look on Sid's face. Sid looked less puzzled and began to smile and show his enjoyment whilst managing to engage in the exercise.

A similar shared and enjoyable response for all three residents continued when hoops were used to introduce certain upper-body exercises. The residents held a hoop in each hand whilst following instruction on making movements with the hoops to increase arm, hand, shoulder and chest movement.

The observation showed a significant increase in all three men's wellbeing levels throughout the 45-minute session. Each of the residents showing increased levels of enjoyment, concentration and engagement with the exercises.

Summary

Using the observational tool allowed me to have measurable evidence of when the residents' wellbeing levels were changing and this identified times when something significant may have been happening within the residents' environment which may influence their levels of wellbeing. A general observation of all residents within the exercise group and their personal response to exercise within that environment provided me with a window to look at some of the physical activity that occurred within the three homes whilst identifying the overall wellbeing of the residents.

I took into account different physical-exercise delivery approaches, one which was based on formal training for staff in care homes, two different outside agencies providing activity and support in care homes, and a less formal approach to engaging dementia residents in physical exercise.

As with all activity and meaningful engagement, this did suggest that a resident's individual physical and cognitive abilities may have an impact upon the level of physical exercise they may be able to engage in. I would suggest from my observations that where staff recognise an individual resident's level of reduced engagement, understanding and a level of support will enable the resident to experience an increased ability to connect and enjoy appropriate physical exercise.

Recognising Al Power's seven domains of wellbeing (2014) both enabled me to reflect upon the outcomes of the observations within the homes and identified for me that physical exercise for residents living with dementia may increase an individual resident's wellbeing. Below are some observational reflections for each of the domains:

- *Identity:* The exercise therapists and staff referred to the residents by name and spoke to all of the individual residents when inviting them to join the physical exercise programme.

- *Connectedness:* Engagement with each individual and sharing the exercise experience with each individual resident occurred regularly. Each person delivering the physical exercise programme spent time to encourage and engage with the resident by offering reassurance and recognising success with the achievements of each individual resident.

- *Security:* Residents were allowed to engage at their own pace and supported to manage their pace and level of involvement without the resident feeling any embarrassment or isolation from the shared experience. Staff who are recognised by residents are important in the delivery of the programme and in supporting the activity. Increased staff presence at the end of the sessions also allows for enjoyment to be shared between staff and residents.

- *Autonomy:* Residents who wish to experience the activity in a unique way are allowed freedom of expression. This includes singing out loud, singing to their choice of music, dancing alone and being expressive in a different form to the programme exercises.

- *Meaning:* Residents become involved in the choice of music and engage with important aspects of their lives such as dancing, conducting with batons, and footballs.

- *Growth:* When playing Bocha, improvement on previous ability and recognition of individual residents' achievement are important, as is the experience of competing against others in a new game.

- *Joy:* Joy was shared by most residents throughout the general observations taken with all the physical exercise sessions. Residents were seen to smile, laugh and become highly involved.

Physical exercise, no doubt, is accepted to have many benefits for an individual's overall health and wellbeing, and a regular programme of physical exercise is regarded as a way to keep active and fit. The individual's level of physical capability does have a proportionate influence on how well the body achieves and maintains the fitness level.

Within the observation, the residents chosen all had different physical and cognitive abilities. The residents' responses were recorded during periods of exercise offered in three different settings and with a variation in the way the exercise was delivered and the gender and age of those delivering the activity. Some residents were able to engage well and accordingly their wellbeing levels were increased easily, whereas other residents took longer to engage and required support and encouragement to experience a short time of increased wellbeing levels.

Residents who were in receipt of the armchair exercise had the opportunity to share an enjoyable and uplifting activity enabling a lot of shared interaction, laughter and joyfulness, and I would suggest that the majority fully took up that opportunity and that physical exercise was seen to be enjoyable and raise their levels of wellbeing. From my perspective, I know my wellbeing levels were increased by sharing these lovely uplifting experiences with our residents.

7

The ImaginationGYM®

LEON SMITH

✳

This chapter explores the therapeutic use of guided visualisation to help residents relax, explore and reminisce in a guided and meaningful way, all without the need to leave the home environment. Research tells us that having access to an external environment is vitally important for physical and mental well-being, but many people living with dementia may find this activity no longer available to them as their physical and mental health diminishes.

The world of reality has its limits; the world of the imagination is boundless.

Jean-Jacques Rousseau

Guided meditation is nothing new and has proven benefits for psychological well-being. However, the activity team at Knightsbridge Care Village in Republic of Ireland have further enhanced this experience by including essential oils along with physical objects such as leaves, flowers and fabrics. We believe we can build on these sessions further by including an element of reminiscence to the visualisation and, as such, the home is currently looking at developing an imaginary 'Walk down our local high street' to allow the person to remember their local community.

These sessions have helped those individuals who sometimes find communal environments both intimidating and noisy. Equally, they allow the person to explore their own reality in a safe and therapeutic way and use the most powerful tools we will ever own in our lifetime: our own brain, life experiences and imagination.

Within this chapter, I would like to explore what makes an activity meaningful to a person living with dementia; after all, we may have all the resources available to put together an activity but if that activity is not appropriate or it doesn't meet the specific needs of the individual then it will more than likely fail to be interesting or stimulating.

I am often sceptical of 'buying into' one form of activity programme and feel that the skill in offering meaningful activity should be flexible and dynamic. There are several ways to assess the level of meaningful activity for a person living with dementia but the most obvious way is 'try it' and see if it works. This is not of course very scientific, but the fun is in the trying and this often offers a level of variety and spontaneity. However, there is a big risk that the person themselves may become despondent – or worse, distressed – if the activity has no meaning to them personally.

Another way to engage our residents is to base an activity upon the individuals' past hobbies and interests or to get family and friends to suggest activities that the person would like. This can really help as it builds on the principles of a good life story (see Chapter 1) and experiences; however, it does not allow for the person to experience new activities and skills.

Preparing for the gym!

Last year, I was invited to join the ImaginationGYM® session at Knightsbridge Care Home. The session was facilitated by the activity co-ordinator Jackie and included ten residents from the Memory Lane Community at the home. The care home has designated specialist areas that are designed to meet the unique and often complex needs of those people living with dementia. Many of the people living within the community have different types of dementia and are likely to be at different stages in their dementia journey. The Memory Lane Community is just that: a community. The staff team, residents and their families play an equal part in their community, with the focus on the person rather than their dementia.

I was initially struck by the planning and attention to detail that Jackie had put into the session before the residents actually arrived. Jackie explained that she liked to set the room up so everyone could see each other and arranged the chairs in a semi-circle. A blanket was placed on each chair, the curtains drawn slightly and the lights turned down rather than off completely. Jackie went to great lengths to ensure each resident was comfortable and that each chair was located in the correct position within the room for each individual person. There was fruit and other food items around the room as well as tea, coffee and water available. Jackie then produced a container with a spray attachment and began spraying the room, chairs and blankets with a mixture of water and essential oils. All this preparation was carried out before anyone set foot in the room.

At this point, all the residents started to arrive and took up their preferred location within the room. The residents taking part in this session were at differing levels of cognitive and physical ability, therefore some residents arrived in wheelchairs whilst others made their own way into the room and a few were accompanied by staff or a family member.

Everyone seemed to be ready to take part and surprisingly I didn't witness one request to leave the room prior to the start of the session.

My experience

In my personal experience as a former carer, I was very aware that starting any group session could be difficult, as many people living with dementia can start to feel anxious as more people enter the room, and there is often a request to leave or go to the toilet. In this session this was not the case and I knew at this point that the activity was something special to all the residents and staff involved.

Jackie started off by making sure everyone was comfortable and the guided visualisation began with the soft sounds of a forest followed by the voice of the lady narrator that took us all on a guided journey through the forest. The room fell silent as we listened to the gentle sounds and I was then able to really focus on the guided imagery. I felt my breathing slowing down as I started to embrace the music and internal images in my mind. I didn't want to close my eyes at this point as I wanted to observe the reactions of the other people in the room. But I could feel the relaxed and calm atmosphere slowly taking effect. I guess the combination of the guided imagery and the collective acceptance from everyone in the room made me feel less self-conscious and allowed me to take full part in this activity. I sat back in my chair, put down my note book and allowed the visions of the forest to form in my mind. In complete honesty, I was initially sceptical that this type of activity would hold the attention of the resident group and wondered when the first request for the toilet or to leave the room would occur. Ten minutes in and yet no one had made a move and 15 minutes later the room still remained full with everyone truly immersed in their own personal journey through the imaginary forest. This was the case until the end of the session and I was truly surprised at how engaged people were in the activity and how relaxed everyone appeared.

However, it is apparent from my observations that for the people in the room that day, it was a welcome break from the hustle and bustle of a modern care home and the anxieties and distress that living in a communal environment might bring.

Introducing poetry

Now that everyone was suitably relaxed and the sense of well-being was now balanced throughout the room, Jackie took centre stage and read out a selection of poems. Most residents were happy to sit and listen; however, there were a few people who knew some of the lines and joined in. Lifelong memories of recalling lines of poetry at school were stimulated and some individuals were transported back to their early years.

Those who did not join in with the recital talked amongst themselves about the poetry or their school years, or just had a general conversation. Again no one asked to leave.

The session finished with a song from one of the residents; this is Ireland, after all, so the link to traditional Irish music is very strong and it wasn't long before everyone joined in.

So why did this session work?

So what magical powers did Jackie have over the individuals within the room? Were they bribed or coerced into staying? Or is there a more scientific or clinical reason for the success of this session? First let's go back to the ImaginationGYM and see what they say about their product and why it works as a therapy.

The ImaginationGYM

The ImaginationGYM is just about going into your imagination and creating stories in your mind, and then bringing some of those ideas back to the real world through a creative endeavour such as storytelling, art, writing, photography, video, drama and so on.

The ImaginationGYM and activity therapy for older people

The ImaginationGYM methodology has been enhanced as it was felt a wider-ranging resource was required to provide a holistic 'Activity Therapy for Older People' in the elder care homes. These modifications were brought about by working directly with staff and residents in the elder care environment. The basic ImaginationGYM Activity Therapy for Older People methodology is focused on imagination exercises, creative activities and a set of rules and principles in the way that the methodology is implemented. The imagination exercises are audio based and designed to stimulate the listener in multiple ways. Not everybody is stimulated in the same way because each person is different but the multiple layers designed into the exercises usually provide some sort of positive stimulation for everyone. This has also proven to be the case in elder care homes.

The activities are designed to encourage participants in the practice of bringing ideas generated in the imaginative state into the real world in practical activities such as drawing, writing, digital media output and so on. It is in this area that most modifications have been made to suit the diversity amongst residents and their individual requirements. When participants are coming from a relaxed imaginative state very often the creative output can be enhanced, or in more difficult circumstances responses can improve (ImaginationGYM 2016).

Unique?

The ImaginationGYM seems to be unique as there is very little research that I can find into the use of meditation/

visualisation for people actually living with dementia. There are several studies into the therapeutic use of meditation for care givers as well as the use of these techniques for people wishing to reduce the risk of cognitive decline. I wanted to establish what research has been published in the therapeutic use of visualisation and mindfulness for people living with dementia and explore how this could be further developed to help individuals to cope with distress and anxiety. Equally I wanted to look at the possibility of stimulating positive memories and to incorporate reminiscence into the visualisation process.

Gard, Holzel and Lazar (2014) suggest that meditation can offset age-related cognitive decline. Studies involved a wide variety of meditation techniques and reported preliminary positive effects on attention, memory, executive function, processing speed and general cognition. Xiong and Doraiswamy (2009) also suggest that meditation practices have various health benefits including the possibility of preserving cognition and preventing dementia. Whilst the mechanisms remain investigational, studies show that meditation may affect multiple pathways that could play a role in brain ageing and mental fitness.

So we know that meditation, visualisation and relaxation techniques have a health benefit for the brain – what other techniques are available, and do they offer any benefit to a person living with dementia?

Mindfulness and other techniques

Mindfulness is about maintaining a moment-by-moment awareness of our thoughts, feelings, bodily sensations and surrounding environment. Mindfulness is thought to have its roots in Buddhist meditation, and studies have shown that practising mindfulness can bring a variety of physical, psychological and social benefits. There is much positive research in the use of mindfulness to reduce stress and how it helps people to cope and improve their relationship with the world around them. Unfortunately there is very little research or evidence that I can find that this could help people living with dementia.

The intervention practice of the 'Kirtan-Kriya' exercise or practices derived from Zen (mantras, breathing exercises in seated meditation positions, visualisation, etc.) are also showing their usefulness in improving cognition and decreasing psychopathology in older people with mild Alzheimer's disease (Moss et al. 2012). These practices seem to produce different health benefits in ageing which are potentially beneficial for the management of institutionalised elderly people in social and healthcare services. Xiong and Doraiswamy (2009) listed the following aspects which indicate the use of these techniques in this population:

- a reduction in cortisol secretion induced by stress, which could have neuroprotective effects by increasing the levels of the brain-derived neurotropic factor

- lipid and oxidative stress reduction, which could reduce the risk of cerebrovascular disease and the neurodegeneration derived from it

- strengthening of the neural circuits and maintenance of the cognitive reserve.

In the same vein, Larouche, Hudon and Goulet (2015) indicate that the practice of mindfulness could slow down cognitive decline, minimising the effects of the symptoms associated with dementia, promoting stress management, reducing the effects of mood disorder and reducing the inflammatory processes associated with neuronal death.

Despite all of this evidence which seems to support the use of these practices, the mechanisms underlying the functioning of mindfulness are still in the research phase (Tang, Hölzel and Posner 2015), and further research into these practices is encouraged.

Reminiscence

The use of reminiscence and life story is the cornerstone of good dementia care, and the importance of gathering and capturing an individual's life experience and memories is starting to shape the ways we can provide meaningful dementia care; however, we could do more.

Su, Wu and Lin (2012) carried out a randomised controlled trial of a six-week spiritual reminiscence intervention on hope, life satisfaction and spiritual well-being in elderly people with mild and moderate dementia. The study identified that hope, life satisfaction and spiritual well-being of elderly patients with mild or moderate dementia could significantly be improved with a six-week spiritual reminiscence intervention.

All this research is important as it continually identifies the therapeutic need for mediation and reminiscence work for people living with dementia; however, it stops short of pulling together the principles of mindfulness, meditation and reminiscence. This is where I feel the ImaginationGYM has further scope to improve. Jackie successfully combined the use of sensory elements such as essential oils and music whilst using the visualisation meditation of the ImaginationGYM CD (ImaginationGYM 2016).

Assessing the need for meaningful activity

Pool (2008a, 2008b) identifies four independent stages of activity. I have used these stages to demonstrate how this guided meditation fits within this model.

Planned activity

An individual is able to work towards completing activities but may not be able to solve any problems that arise in the process. During the ImaginationGYM session some individuals were able to follow the visualisation and the instructions given by Jackie but struggled when the verbal language became too complex. It was good to see how naturally Jackie and her team were able to identify this and adjust how they communicated with the people in the room. This skill comes from knowing your residents and can't be easily taught, so for the ImaginationGYM session to be successful you must first know your resident group.

Exploration

The individual is now less concerned with consequences of carrying out the activity and may not have an end result in mind but is able to carry out familiar activities in familiar surroundings. The ImaginationGYM is very much about exploration, both on a physical level such as touching and feeling objects around you as well as mentally exploring an environment using the visualisation techniques. The majority of the individuals taking part in the imagination session were responding at this level.

Sensory

An individual may now only respond to sensation and only be able to carry out single-step activities such as touch, listening and watching. For those people with this level of activity Jackie was very careful not to overload the person: they were allowed the time and space to listen to the guided visualisation, enjoy their drink or watch others in the room. It was interesting how music, singing and poetry had a positive effect for those individuals at this level of cognition.

Reflex

Some individuals may not be aware of the surrounding environment or their own body, and therefore need direct sensory stimulation to raise self-awareness. It is important not to overstimulate or use multiple stimuli at one time, therefore a crowded and noisy environment could be problematic. It may seem initially that the ImaginationGYM would be inappropriate for an individual at this level of activity, but I observed several residents who had very little awareness of their surroundings and were not appearing to listen to the visualisation narrative but were happy to be in the room, sharing their space with other people. I felt this was more like a non-verbal bonding experience that was not overchallenging to the individual. I was expecting more individuals who would be assessed at a reflex level to find the ImaginationGYM too slow and not stimulating; however, this was not the case and they stayed until the end of the session.

Pool (2008a) recognised that people with cognitive impairment have potential abilities that can be realised when in an enabling environment, and that occupation is the key to unlocking this potential.

So why is the ImaginationGYM important?

People living with dementia can experience symptoms of distress as part of their condition as well as other symptoms such as restlessness and depression. There are many reasons a person living with dementia may become distressed, including infections, loss of life skills, embarrassment and stress on relying on others to care for them, and so on. However, (without training) staff may still rely on drug therapies to treat these episodes of distress. The Alzheimer's Society offers very helpful guidelines on appropriate approaches to managing and supporting people who become distressed. In relation to the use of activity particularly, some of these include:

- engaging the person in enjoyable and meaningful activities

- spending quality time with the person

- ensuring that they build up social networks and feel included

- sharing activities with others, which may promote shared interest and increase interactions and understanding

- having a relaxing atmosphere to help the person to feel calm and secure.

Helping residents to feel secure is so important especially when living in a communal environment. Distress is often caused by external demands and pressures, so any opportunity to get away from these pressures can be really important for a person living with dementia. The ImaginationGYM allows the person to be in control of their environment and free from noise and distraction. It allows the person to socialise with others and be part of the home community in a way that is not overwhelming or overstimulating. Equally, the staff team have a forum where they can sit with a person and get to really know and understand their life story, beliefs, wishes and aspirations. I feel the ImaginationGYM should be part of a strategy in helping people living with dementia to reduce their level of distress and anxiety. This activity offers a more natural and person-centred approach to tackling distress and can avoid the more conventional medical interventions.

The state of being comfortable, healthy or happy

Power (2014), in his book *Dementia Beyond Disease*, argues that people with dementia are not psychotic or delusional; rather, they see the world differently than others. He also goes on to define the seven domains of well-being and again we can see how this model fits in with the principles of the ImaginationGYM.

- *Identity:* Jackie took great care in making sure everyone knew each other and that the individual needs for the person were in place right at the beginning. Items such as blankets, empathy dolls and other personalised objects were placed on the chairs prior to the residents entering the room. This level of detail helped to make the person feel they were personally involved in the whole experience; additionally it was nice to see family members accompanying their loved one to this session.

- *Connectedness:* It appeared that all of the people attending the ImaginationGYM session were connected, which was very evident in the general conversation within the room, and this soon turned into mutual reflective silence followed by the collective singing at the end of the session. Jackie informed me that residents, staff and family members all enjoyed getting involved within the ImaginationGYM as it bought them together as a community.

- *Security:* Everyone was asked at the beginning of the session if they were comfortable and if they were happy to proceed with the session. No one was coerced into taking part, and when necessary, residents could leave the session without fear or anxiety. Jackie had ensured that the right mix of residents were together for companionship.

- *Autonomy:* All residents were given a choice of attending this session; they were also given the choice as to where to sit. Both food and drink choices were offered, and any requests were dealt with straight away. The level of control for the individual didn't stop after the ImaginationGYM session; each resident was given the opportunity to choose their favourite poem or to sing their favourite song. There was a level of mutual respect for people's wishes and there was very little evidence of conflict.

- *Meaning:* As explained earlier in this chapter, the need for meaningful activity is so important to reduce episodes of distress and anxiety as well as promoting well-being. As there were no incidents of distress reaction at any point during the session I felt that this was a good indication of the well-being level within the room. Many residents had returned to this activity on many occasions, which also demonstrated that they found this session meaningful.

- *Growth:* I have discussed the importance of reminiscence work and the need to tap into past memories; however, the ImaginationGYM also allowed the residents to experience something different. Guided visualisation would probably not have been available to many of the residents during their earlier years; many residents felt that they had learnt a lot about themselves and they had reconnected with long-forgotten memories.

- *Joy:* The level of joy, happiness and mutual acceptance of others was really evident during the singing at the end of the session. It felt to me that after all the quiet, reflective guided meditation, singing was a sort of mutual release of positive energy. I feel our appreciation of music and singing so often comes from our emotions. It is not important to actually know the words or be able to play the music; it is more a way of letting out and sharing our emotions. This was very much the case in this session: the singing was a validation of our well-being and we were not afraid to show it!

Summary

The ImaginationGYM offers a lot more than simply guided visualisation, as it's perhaps more about the opportunity to relax and reflect. Many people living with dementia can experience a high level of anxiety and may find the world around them moving too fast, and then it becomes very easy to disconnect yourself from the world. This session, however, I felt gave everybody the chance to collectively connect with the people around us. It also brings residents, care givers and family members together. It gives you the opportunity to let go of anxiety and to focus on the positive. The activity allows the individual to reminisce and to remember those forgotten memories from the earlier years, plus it offers the chance to experience something new and to grow in a creative way.

For me it was fun! I really enjoyed being part of the group and sharing their positive energy and laughter. I feel this type of guided meditation has a real place in care home environments and I feel it would benefit residents, their families and the staff team. It is important to remember that group activities do not need to be grandiose affairs involving external entertainers at large expense to the home. They can be inexpensive with minimal staff input. They can be meaningful and expressive without the need for costly specialist equipment. There is no need for specially trained staff, just regular staff members who know their residents very well. It's an activity that everyone can participate in, including family members and outsiders like me. It was a privilege to be part of this activity and I look forward to joining the Memory Lane Community at Knightsbridge Care Home again soon.

Memory has thousands of eyes staring into the experiences of the past, while imagination peers into every corner of the universe.

James Lendall Basford,
Seven Seventy Seven Sensations (1897)

8

Creativity

Incorporating Activity into Everyday Life

DEENA HEANEY

❋

This chapter will introduce interventions which support activity being incorporated into everyday life in the care home. The author demonstrates that by getting to know residents, understanding their life story and working with residents, families and care staff, meaningful activity can be offered to encourage independence whilst providing the opportunity for participation which enhances the residents' well-being.

What is activity?

Activity is defined as 'a situation in which something is happening or a lot of things are being done' (Oxford Learner's Dictionaries 2017). Activity has potential in that it's an opportunity to create a moment that means something in everything we do. Involvement in activity will depend upon the needs and abilities of individuals and the resources available; however, everyday life can provide many opportunities for individuals to undertake activity.

Residents will enjoy a variety of interests. Group activity is beneficial for some residents. The joining together to enjoy a social occasion and reminiscing can promote positive memory and give residents the opportunity to share their experiences, which enhances communication. Arts and crafts provide the opportunity for residents to be creative, as well as singing and dancing and generally having fun. Outings to different places of interest such as the local coffee shop help maintain connections with the residents' local community. Residents will often enjoy individual activity, for example, reading a book or a newspaper (either reading on their own or someone reading to them). A hand massage or a makeover can also be relaxing and the physical touch can provide comfort for the person participating. Physical activity such as walking, armchair exercise, dancing and playing bowls will all support physical and emotional well-being.

NICE guidelines (2013) state that it is important that older people in care homes have the opportunity to take part in activity, including activities of daily living, that helps to maintain or improve their health and mental well-being. They should be encouraged to take an active role in choosing and defining activities that are meaningful to them. Whenever possible, and if the person wishes, family, friends and carers should be involved in these activities. This will help to ensure that activity is meaningful and that relationships are developed and maintained.

Most of the care homes in the company we work for employ activity coordinators. Part of their role is to develop, implement and participate in activity along with staff on a daily and weekly basis. In this chapter, we are going to focus on daily activity – things that we all do most days that we may not consider to be an activity, but which have an overall positive sense of remaining involved in 'normal' things. Some of the most beneficial activities can be simple: everyday tasks such as setting the table for a meal or folding clothes. Activities such as these can help a person living with dementia to feel connected to normal life and can enhance autonomy, identity, a sense of purpose and ultimately well-being.

The resident

So, what do we know about the resident? Each unique individual we support has their own full, rich life story (see Chapter 1). The residents' likes and dislikes, significant relationships in their lives, previous occupations and hobbies and interests are so important to help us to provide meaningful activities for the resident to participate in. Our staff complete the Getting to Know Me Books with the resident and their family and friends to record significant information. When asking the right questions and, more importantly, listening intently to the answers, we will create a picture of the resident's life, otherwise known as their 'life story'. Once we have a clear understanding of the person's life story, we are better equipped to fulfil their current stage of life and well-being with meaningful activity.

If a resident is living with dementia their reality may be different to ours. It is therefore essential we respect this and validate their feelings by stepping into their reality. For example, a resident may believe they are much younger than they actually are and may be telling you they need to go to work. The resident may be trying to express that they need to feel useful and valued, as they once did when they went to work. Involving the resident in daily living activity will support the person's feelings and fulfil needs. According to Naomi Feil (2015), 'to validate is to acknowledge the feelings of a person. To validate someone is to say that his or her feelings are true. Denying feelings invalidates the individual' (p.14).

Allow me to explain with a case study. This case study emphasises the importance of understanding not only Gladys, but any individual you are supporting to achieve their potential, whilst respecting their reality.

Gladys has lived at the home for 16 months. Gladys enjoys walking around the home with her duster and cleans the handrails, pictures and ornaments whilst on her walks.

The staff know that Gladys once worked as a housekeeper in a stately home. Gladys enjoys her 'work' and chats with other residents whilst carrying out her tasks.

During a support visit to the home, I bid Gladys a 'good morning' and enquired as to how she was. Gladys' response was, 'Well, I'm all right but I'm going to be leaving here soon; I have had enough. I work hard to keep the place clean and I know they give me a room and food but if I were you I wouldn't come and work here because they don't pay you. I have worked here for years and they never give me a penny.' Gladys then walked away chuntering and swearing. Staff told me this is a daily occurrence; however, the staff did not really recognise this as distress. I discussed with staff the importance of not only validating Gladys' feelings, as she was obviously upset about not getting paid for her work (wouldn't you be upset if you didn't receive your wages?!), but also the need to respect Gladys' reality.

Due to the progression of her dementia, Gladys perceived herself to be 32 years old. In considering Gladys' life story and respecting her reality, at 32 years old she would have been employed as a housekeeper who lived in at her job but also received a wage. Therefore it makes perfect sense to Gladys that she should be receiving a wage for her work, and she is justified in feeling annoyed and communicating her feelings.

I met with Gladys' son and he explained that his mother constantly talks about leaving her 'job' due to not being paid. Although he respects her reality, giving her reassurance that he looks after her money and that she can have money whenever she wants, he finds the situation difficult to support. We felt that Gladys understands what money is; however, she no longer understood the value of money. We discussed, therefore, that the amount of money she would be paid was not important, but the principle of receiving some money for her work was. Following a risk assessment (the money could be lost or mislaid), Gladys' son agreed he would purchase some wage packets and put £6.00 of change in once a week, which he would then put through the administrator's door each Thursday evening when he visited, and Gladys would be informed pay day would be on a Friday. This information was disseminated to the staff team, which ensured a consistent approach when communicating with Gladys. Gladys was told that pay day was every Friday and was reminded of this when asking for her wages.

I visited the home a few weeks later and Gladys was walking round with her duster cleaning pictures and chatting to other residents. I asked Gladys how she was and she told me she was 'too busy to talk' to me as she had 'work to do' and happily went about her duties! Staff commented how they were now able to respond to Gladys positively – 'Payday is on Friday and it's Wednesday today, so only two more days' – resulting in communication being effective and minimising Gladys' distress.

The staff

Whilst care for any individual can sometimes be complex, it is a skilful and ultimately rewarding role. The common misconception is that carers do not have the time to support residents in their chosen activity, and ultimately activity only takes place when the activity coordinator is on duty. Helping staff to understand that activity is anything and everything we do is really important. As a dementia care support team, we have written several training courses to support staff understanding: not only of the diagnosis of dementia but also of a person-centred approach to dementia care. Bespoke courses have also been developed, one of which includes 'understanding activity and meaningful occupation'. This course helps staff to understand different types of activity and how we can support and encourage residents to be involved, especially in daily living activity, based on the knowledge we have of a person's life story.

Brooker (2007, p.109) states that, 'If people feel enabled to do things rather than prevented from following their desires, they are more likely to be in a state of better emotional well-being over time.' It is not my view that staff intentionally set out to 'de-skill' residents by doing everything for them. I genuinely think that staff often believe that by doing everything for residents, their practice demonstrates that they care. Educating staff to better understand how to support residents with activities that are meaningful can provide various benefits including enhancing a sense of purpose to fulfil a physical or emotional need, understanding what the resident's preferences are, what they are still able to do independently and what areas they may need support with. All of these can build upon and promote positive relationships. Helping people to feel connected will ultimately give staff the confidence to practise different approaches, and involving the residents in the task and utilising the residents' skills will become normal practice.

Of course, in order to prevent setting a person up to fail, we must not only ensure the opportunity offered is an appropriate activity to meet their need, but also consider the person's changing ability due to the progression of their illness. We would therefore utilise Jackie Pool's Activity Level documentation. Pool (2012, pp.54–55) states that, 'In order to present an occupation to the person with cognitive impairment so that he/she can engage with it, his/her impairment and abilities must be first understood.' Utilising the Pool tool helps to define the best way of presenting the activity to the resident, supporting us to identify the level of ability in order to ensure success.

I would like to demonstrate in this chapter that by understanding the definition of activity and the different types of activity, we will become more confident in offering the opportunity for residents to participate in daily living activity – that is, activity which many residents have probably participated in for much of their life. For example, consider the dining experience. Good nutrition and hydration are essential for life but should be combined to facilitate a pleasant experience we all would enjoy and hope for. Let me elaborate with another case study – meet Gill:

Gill is collecting the plates of other residents who are sitting at her table. (Unfortunately several of them are still eating!) Staff spend much of their time asking Gill to sit down and telling her not to collect the plates as they will do that, and Gill becomes quite annoyed at the staff. Gill may also be labelled as 'a problem' or not compliant with 'routine'. We have learned by understanding her life story that Gill used to work in a school kitchen for 15 years, and every day after serving hundreds of children their meal, she would spend an allotted time collecting crockery from the tables and washing and drying the dishes; and actually she quite misses not only the interaction with her colleagues, but also the process of helping people. So why not provide the opportunity for Gill to participate in this 'activity'? We may have to slightly adapt the activity: perhaps have a few plates ready to be washed to discourage Gill from removing plates when people are still eating – this approach would enable staff to provide acknowledgement of Gill's assistance. For example, we could thank Gill for her help and suggest she washes the plates which are already stacked, before washing the plates of residents who are still eating, as opposed to telling Gill she can't do something.

> Turn this into a positive experience for Gill. Of course we have to consider health and safety, and ultimately the crockery at some point will have to be sterilised in the dishwasher, but denying Gill the opportunity of completing something she can still do which has a positive impact on her well-being will almost certainly affect Gill's sense of purpose, participation, connectedness and sense of achievement. This in turn may contribute to eroding her autonomy, which will have a significant negative impact on her emotional well-being. Power (2014) states that when considering the seven domains of well-being, we can help find ways to safely restore choice and control.

When thinking of ourselves, we wouldn't want to sit and eat at a cluttered dining table, would we? We would want to have a nice place to sit with a clean chair, a clean place mat, a clean plate and clean cutlery. Equally, if we were going to a restaurant, we would probably have an expectation of how that environment would be presented, so why would this be any different for the resident?

I have supported homes where staff bring their own food and sit at the dining table with the residents to eat, making the dining experience a real social opportunity, whilst at other homes staff choose from the menu and sit with the residents as a planned activity. Chatting and eating together, getting to know each other and enjoying each other's company have had a positive effect on residents, enhancing their autonomy and connectedness and increasing well-being.

Family and friends

Never underestimate the importance of family and friends. These people are the residents' nearest and dearest and will help you, as we have learned, to understand the individuals' life stories.

The diagnosis of dementia does not only affect the person diagnosed: dementia can also have a negative (sometimes massive) impact on a resident's family and friends. In my experience of working with families and friends, they often speak of the loss of the person they once knew, the loss of a future they had planned together and the difficulty in communicating with their loved one due to the way in which the person now communicates. Families and friends will need support in not only understanding the diagnosis of dementia, but also how they can remain a constant support in their loved one's life. Enjoying activity together can be fun and it supports identity, security and connectedness – three of the seven domains of well-being identified by Power (2014). Family and friends in general are only too pleased to participate in activities with their loved ones and to play a pivotal role, especially with group activities, such as open days or afternoon parties.

Continuing the focus on daily living activity, my next case study will demonstrate the sense of fulfilment for Nancy (who used to be a housewife) in continuing to provide, as she has always done, for her family.

Nancy has lived at the care home for six months and she is living with frontotemporal dementia. Nancy has three daughters and a son. Nancy's family visit her most days. Nancy really looks forward to seeing her family and spends much of her day waiting for her family to visit. During visits, they spend time in Nancy's room chatting, which can result in the room becoming a little overcrowded. Nancy often becomes distressed as she can't always relate to the conversations taking place in her room. This in turn causes the family to become upset. Staff attempt to find an alternative larger space in the home for Nancy to spend time with her family; however, this can prove difficult at times, especially if other residents go into the room, as Nancy shouts at other residents to 'Get out of my house!'

During one particular visit, the chef had made some cakes and Nancy and her family were offered tea and cakes. Nancy said they were nice, but not nearly as nice as the ones she used to make. This led to Nancy and her family reminiscing about the hours of fun they had baking cakes together then sitting round the kitchen table sampling their efforts!

The care home had a 'living skills' kitchen which provided the opportunity for residents to participate by making drinks, washing up, wiping surfaces, and all the usual everyday things that we all do as part of our daily lives. One of Nancy's daughters asked staff if they could use the kitchen to bake some cakes with their mum and this was agreed. On their next visit, two of Nancy's daughters brought ingredients to bake cakes and set to work with Nancy in baking a cake. The daughters were really surprised at how positively their mum involved herself in the experience. They had noticed a rapid decline in their mother's ability to do what they considered to be simple everyday tasks, but she certainly showed great skill in making the cake, recalling which ingredients were to be added. Once the cake was ready to eat, Nancy and her family sat at the table enjoying their hard work! Nancy's family were delighted and expressed how uplifting it was for them as well as their mother to do something 'normal' together: something they would have ordinarily done when spending time with their mother before she had moved to live in the care home. The family continue to bake with Nancy at least once a month. This activity has supported them all in meaningful communication and enhanced connectedness.

The environment

So, why is the environment important? A person living with dementia does not always interpret their environment the same way as you or me. The more opportunity we provide for the residents to participate in daily living activity, the greater the chance of enhancing independence and well being. Baker (2015) explains that the key focus within any dementia care environment is to try to make it as relaxed and calm as possible. We should also give consideration to other aspects of the environment: it should be stimulating (for those who wish to seek out activity), homely, enabling and orientating (see Chapter 9).

- *Stimulating:* The environment should be object-rich with interesting things to do and see along the resident's chosen route. Different fabrics/textiles to stimulate sensory need (hats, scarves, etc.), and rummage boxes containing interesting items for the resident to see and touch – can lead to positive effective communication – residents having the opportunity to take things out of the rummage box which may promote positive memories.

- *Homely:* It should contain age-appropriate furniture and items which would appear familiar to residents, and be comfortable and not clinical; chairs in communal lounges should not be placed round the edge of the room but be arranged in small groups which will encourage socialisation. (It's more likely the resident will join a small group rather than a big open group – it could be quite a daunting experience if you are not a very confident person to walk into a room full of strangers and be expected to sit with everyone.) Placing chairs in smaller groups also affords the opportunity of a variety of different activities being available, promoting choice for the residents.

- *Enabling:* It should have sufficient rest areas in corridors and public areas, ensuring the individual can complete their journey without getting tired, or utilise the corridor for somewhere to sit quietly on their own.

- *Orientating:* There should be clear signage for direction which can support orientation and minimise confusion, on bedroom doors, bathroom doors, communal lounges and dining rooms, and in themed corridors.

Washing clothes and hanging them out to dry may seem a mundane task to us, but if that's a skill you can still accomplish, it's an achievement!

In my next case study, meet Doris:

Doris likes to walk round the environment. She always has her shopping bag with her and collects lots of different items along the way, but in particular likes to collect clothes, scarves and fabrics. Doris will often tell staff she is worried the children's clothes are not clean and needs to get them washed – Doris is a mother to eight children! The staff have offered to take the clothes to the laundry and get them washed. However, Doris is reluctant to part with her collection as she is concerned the children will have nothing to wear. With the support of staff, Doris has been encouraged to wash the clothes in the sink in the living skills kitchen, and a clothes line has also been purchased for Doris and the staff to hang out clothes together. Doris takes great delight in folding the clothing once it is dry, gaining tremendous satisfaction in a job well done!

Benefit of daily living activity

What would you like the residents to achieve? Are they able to achieve this? Are you providing opportunities for residents to be involved in daily living activity?

Our understanding of the resident through their life story and having a clear knowledge of their interests, their hobbies, their work, their relationships, their family and their friends all significantly contribute to helping the resident not only participate in something that they enjoy but also feel a sense of control, ownership or pride.

Rather than a generic activity, we need to focus on what the resident enjoys and perhaps what they miss. No matter how simple (or perhaps boring) you think the activity is, if it is the resident's choice and you can observe a real sense of interaction, engagement or pleasure then the resident should be encouraged to continue. The important ingredient to any activity is not setting the resident up to fail. By that I mean it should be an activity that they enjoy and can accomplish with a sense of pride and achievement, and they should not be encouraged to do something that they can no longer do, which can leave them feeling deflated or with no sense of purpose.

Until his physical health deteriorated, Frank rented an allotment. My next case study demonstrates how a little bit of imagination can enhance a person's well-being:

Frank has lived at the home for two years and is living with vascular dementia. During a support visit, staff spoke to me of how they were finding it difficult to support Frank as he often seemed to be angry and no matter how they tried to support him, he always appeared annoyed with them. He has lost the ability to speak and communicates by using gestures, such as pushing staff away or turning away from staff when they are attempting to support him. Frank has no family and receives no visitors. It has therefore been quite difficult for staff to identify Frank's life story. They do know, however, that Frank loves to sit outside in his wheelchair admiring the garden, and they ensure he spends as much time as possible outdoors. If there are weeds which haven't been pulled out or leaves that have not been cleared, obscuring the view of the flowerbeds, Frank attempts to lean out of his wheelchair to try to rectify the situation. Staff engage with Frank by asking him to show them what needs to be done and which flowers need attention. I suggested that Frank may be communicating negatively due to not being able to carry out tasks he once enjoyed and was successful at achieving.

A raised garden bed has been created for Frank. This is at an appropriate height to enable him access whilst he is in his wheelchair. Staff spent time with Frank looking through different gardening books to support him in choosing what he would like to grow in his 'mini-allotment'. Frank gestured that he would like to create a vegetable garden, and was taken to the local garden centre to purchase the necessary seeds and then began working on his creation. Frank has grown some wonderful vegetables which he is really proud of. The chef will often help him pick the vegetables and cook them to accompany his meal. Staff can now engage positively with Frank and often share their gardening failures with him. Seeking his advice both demonstrates respect in valuing Frank's opinion and expertise and enhances his autonomy.

Maintaining the well-being of the individual

We have covered several aspects of activity throughout this chapter; a positive result is only achievable once we understand the uniqueness of the individual we are supporting. The sense of fulfilment and satisfaction will not only be felt by the resident but also by the staff working alongside the resident, as together with colleagues and the resident's family and friends, we will have enabled the resident to accomplish an activity that they enjoy, they miss but can still participate in.

Summary

Research clearly evidences that when activity is incorporated into everyday life, residents' well-being is enhanced.

It has been and continues to be a pleasure and privilege, in my 34 years' experience of supporting a person living with dementia, to work with staff, families and friends, observing a resident who is meaningfully occupied. I have felt truly humbled witnessing positive emotional well-being and joy and observing how distress has been minimised through the opportunity for residents to be engaged in daily living activity.

Educating staff in the importance of normal daily living activity in everyday life, understanding the person, adapting activity to meet the changing need and ability whilst offering the opportunity for inclusion – all will enhance a sense of purpose, and support identity and autonomy.

Activity is anything and everything we do. It's not about the result, it's about the taking part: the being involved. Dementia Care Australia (2017) suggests that the true focus is not about the activity itself but the quality and joy of the interaction. Just because someone changes their address doesn't mean they have to change their lifestyle!

In considering the seven domains of well-being (Power 2014), supporting a resident to maintain daily skills enhances their well-being:

- Understanding the resident, getting to know them and offering the opportunity to be involved in daily living activity reinforce *identity*.

- Being involved with others and completing tasks together provides the opportunity for *connectedness*.

- Providing an environment in which residents feel comfortable and at home where they can be involved in completing everyday tasks provides a sense of *security*.

- Offering the opportunity for residents to be involved in daily living activity will support the resident in decision making, enhancing *autonomy*.

- Supporting residents to participate in activity which they have always been involved in gives *meaning*.

- Providing new experiences for daily living activity which a resident may not have previously done will promote *growth*.

- All of the above will ultimately lead to *joy*, celebrating life and living well.

Key tips for implementing daily life skills

- Is it just one resident who enjoys this activity? There may be several residents who enjoy similar activity and this could be a regular thing, bringing more joy to more people, more often.

- Don't forget to involve family and friends who can share their interests and hobbies.

- Get to know the person you are supporting – understand their life story.

- Involve the resident in everyday tasks which will provide the opportunity for daily living activity, such as helping to make the bed, wash the pots, wipe down surfaces or setting dining tables.

- Make every interaction with a resident an opportunity for positive communication.

9

Environments that Can Help to Stimulate or Relax

CAROLINE BAKER AND HOLLY RANCE

✳

This chapter will focus on the key things that can be introduced to help residents not only find their own way around the environment but also participate in meaningful activity independently or with a relative, friend or a member of staff as they make their way around the home.

I was recently asked to present at a conference in Oslo, and it was with some trepidation that I was informed that it was much easier to take the train to the venue from the airport than it was to get a taxi there. The organisers were very helpful and had told me where the train platform usually was and to head for Central Station (Sentralstarjon), and then gave me information as to how to get to the hotel which was 'just across the road'. From there, I would take a taxi to the conference venue itself once I had checked into the hotel. After printing off the information and studying it on the plane, I felt quite confident that this would be easy to achieve, even though it was in a different country and language.

However, when I came out of the airport and followed the signs for the trains, there were two different companies offering two different services and as I scanned all of the information boards, I was unable to locate a train that appeared to go to Central Station and now I began to panic! I approached an employee who had a uniform on (that matched one of the train service logos) and showed her my documentation. She was very helpful and said that I needed to take a particular train that would go through the station that I needed, and she told me the platform number.

Feeling a little more confident, I boarded the train, sitting amongst people who spoke a very different language to me, and began watching a digital screen of adverts and news, also not in English (obviously!). But I began to worry again that I might not know which stop I should get off at, or how long it may be before I needed to disembark, so I sat with my case firmly by my side and my coat still on! It was then that I spotted a 'journey planner' similar to those we have on the trains in England and saw that it was the second stop so at least I knew that once I had gone through one station, the next stop would be the one I needed.

I got off the train and turned right as I had been instructed and walked through the huge station to the other end. As I stood outside scanning the horizon, I was unable to see the hotel that was 'just across the road'. I therefore went back into the station to the other side and, to my relief, saw the hotel that I was booked into. Check-in was very simple and straightforward, the receptionist spoke English and I located and checked into my room. I hung my clothes, grabbed a coffee and then headed out to the taxi rank that was just outside of the hotel. I showed the driver the address that I had and he nodded and whisked me away. At this point, I started to relax! The driver knew where we were going and I would be at the conference door ready to present in an hour.

Unfortunately, there were some significant roadworks around the conference centre and so the taxi driver pulled into a layby and explained that he was unable to get directly outside of the centre, but I just had to cross the road and it was at the back of the building. Simple! I walked round the building twice and couldn't see the name of the conference centre I was due to be at. I tried to recall which road he had taken to try to access the centre, and I walked through scaffolding amidst a cacophony of drills and other noises which began hampering both my tolerance and my thoughts, looking up at each building for a sign that I may be near. I stopped a passer-by, asked if they spoke English (they did!), and asked if they could help me to locate the conference centre, showing them the name that I had written down. They gave me directions which sounded quite simple and I set off with renewed vigour, confident that I would be at my destination very soon. But despite going round and round, I still couldn't locate the venue. I was now very cold, becoming tired and frustrated and wondering if they would actually miss me if I just grabbed a taxi back to the hotel!

At this point, two very charming young gentlemen observed me holding my papers with a perplexed look on my face and asked if I needed any help. I explained what had happened and that I was now in danger of being seriously late, and my knights in shining armour walked with me to show me the way (very person centred!).

The reason for my story here is quite simple. Signage and communication plays such an important part of our lives and can either help or hinder our progress and our internal feelings of confidence and mood. I wonder if this may be how some of our residents feel when trying to navigate their way around our buildings. Do we precipitate increasing frustration (and confusion) if we do not provide appropriate signage or colours to try to help people locate their room or the toilet or where they head to get some food? Far better to increase independence and reduce confusion by trying to make the environment cues as clear as possible.

As part of our programme to enhance dementia care, we looked at papers and guidance from many avenues, but the King's Fund tool (2014) helped enormously in identifying what we already had in place and the measures that we needed to take to improve the environment within the care home. Tilly and Reed (2008) state that in the case of behavioural distress, environmental techniques should be amongst the first strategies used as a treatment, rather than beginning with pharmacologic interventions. If we look back to my introductory tale, I was beginning to become quite distressed, and we have to consider how much of a resident's distress may be due to increased confusion, frustration or overstimulation. The environment consists not only of paint and furnishings but also of the noises and stimuli within a care home: staff shouting across to each other, scraping dinner plates and throwing cutlery into a bowl, call bells, trolleys being pushed across wooden floors and telephones ringing. Along with the physical environment, it is crucial that we educate staff about the impact of heightened stimuli (or indeed lack of stimuli).

Within this chapter we will focus mainly on communal areas, as my colleagues discuss other elements of design within their chapters. We have not followed any guidance by rote but, within the pilot of our programme, tested out things that we thought may work following the general guidance. Some of our homes used different approaches as they were quite different buildings but, ultimately, they all followed a similar colour scheme.

We are very fortunate within the company to have experts in interior design who not only are experienced in helping us with colours and themes but also genuinely listened and understood our concerns around various items that had previously been introduced and were then taken out of the 'pack'. Our interior design staff attended our dementia care training at the beginning of the pilot to enable them to have a greater understanding of how a diagnosis of dementia might impact on a person and their environment in terms of well-being and ill-being.

The design of the physical environment plays a major role in supporting people with dementia. The colours, textures, signage, lighting and overall aesthetics can change, develop and encourage different behaviours and patterns in a person's day-to-day life. Being part of the dementia care programme pilot and linking interior design with other practices has been a real learning curve. It has also provided a great platform to utilise our knowledge and learning from an interior design perspective and also from experiences working in the care environment. This chapter gives an overview of the design we have conceptualised and implemented within some of our homes and also the rationale, philosophy and research behind this.

The use of colour, themes and design
Corridors

Finding one's way easily, safely and with some enjoyment along the way is the key part of successful corridor design. The design of the physical environment plays a major role in supporting the way-finding abilities of people with dementia (Marquardt 2011). When looking at the design of the corridors in our homes, we established that we have such a wide variety of styles, shapes, configurations, light levels and ambience that we needed an approach that would work harmoniously in all. Some corridors are wide and long, others have alcoves, whilst others are very narrow and straight. The challenge was coming up with ideas that would not only successfully guide the residents around but also give them a sense of belonging and understanding in their home.

The first port of call was thinking about the physical factors that make up the corridor: the walls, handrails, doors, corners, ceilings and skirting boards. We looked at the challenges these present and how to enable the key functional elements to stand out. The handrails divide the corridor wall space in two, and therefore create a natural colour break in the paintwork. Research has suggested that older people tend to look downwards (Namazi and Johnson 1991), which links to our decision to paint beneath the rail in the deeper colour, with a neutral colour above in the narrower corridors. This has proven to be successful in our pilot homes as the residents visually follow the colour and utilise it to recognise their bedroom corridor, or perhaps the day space location. The colour differentiation also helps the handrail to stand out, and having a simple wooden bullnose trim brings texture, dimension and an organic homely feel to the corridor. Where some corridors are irregular shapes and are more complex with doors in alcoves, we have used the same colour palette as previously described, but have used 'feature walls' to identify areas instead. This has proven to be equally successful and still has the same look and feel as our original piloted idea.

The paint colours chosen to take the residents on this journey were a selection to match the corridor 'themes' that we have integrated to add some interest to these long spaces. The 'theme packs' provide visual stimulation and are based around activities or interests that the residents may have had or taken part in in their earlier years. A 'less is more' approach means there is a concentrated focus down what could appear as a long uninviting corridor. Each section has its own colour identification and theme, for example the 'garden' corridor has a display unit filled with garden-themed accessories which in turn complements the green paint on the walls (see Figure 9.2). These areas are interactive and the residents are encouraged to touch and move the items, even take them with them around the home. The items are then replenished or returned at the end of the day ready for the next day's adventure. At the next corner, the theme and colour would move on, to help the residents identify they are changing area. The themes are supported with relevant artwork in clear, bold, usually photographic images to provoke memory and add to the overall ambience and aesthetic. Interesting artworks encourage mobility and conversation as well as helping people find their way around (King's Fund 2014).

With the corridors now full of colour, art and accessories, we made the decision to paint the inside of the bedroom doors white. The thinking behind white bedroom doors is both to enhance the coloured signs that are used but also to enable the (coloured) toilet doors within the corridor to have more prominence. The ironmongery is very obvious and stands out well against the white. The back-of-house doors and cross-corridor doors (Figure 9.1) are painted in the same tones as the corridor, to blend the doors in and make them disappear visually to residents and not distract or distress, as locked doors can lead to frustration and anger when they cannot be opened (King's Fund 2014).

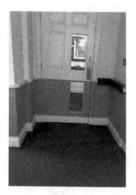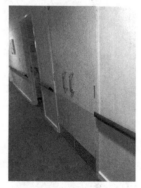

Figure 9.1 Examples of a 'blended door'

Another corridor feature we include in some homes are photographic murals (Figure 9.2). These help with navigation, and also add a point of interest for the residents. The selection of images we have chosen are mainly panoramic, portraying a view of standing on a balcony looking out. The images are in proportion and have no 'over-sized' elements that could cause confusion or anxiety. The aim is for these to blend in with the hues around, but to also add another dimension and visual clue to help the resident as they travel around the space. The visuals provide a talking point, and potentially stimulation of memories for residents, families and visitors alike.

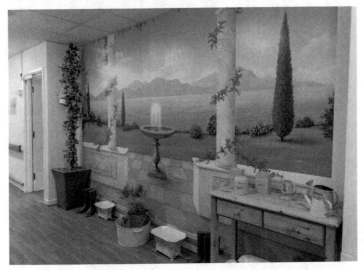

Figure 9.2 Example of a 'garden theme' corridor with mural rather than paint

Signage

One of the key way-finding properties we have developed is our signage collection. We wanted to develop a bedroom sign that incorporated all the elements of research plus our own ideas to create something unique and identifiable. Many people with moderate to severe dementia are able to identify written names and photographs of themselves (Marquardt 2011). We developed a sign that is simple, bold and clear, coloured in the same tones as the corridor so it ties in yet stands out on the white doors. The sign has a section for the resident's name, the room number is embossed and there is a square for a photograph. The sign comes in two sizes, one for traditional six-panel doors, and also a larger A4 size for flat doors. We realised during the trial that we have such a variety of door styles amongst the homes that we needed options. The signs are attached directly onto the doors as it is recommended that signage should be placed *on* doors and not beside them (King's Fund 2014).

We also developed day room signage options. We wanted signage that matched the other ironmongery in the home, so we went for a brushed steel finish. The signs contain the name of the room, and an image that best symbolises the purpose of the space. The writing is simple with upper- and lower-case fonts, yet the signs look upmarket and smart. The images are bold and clear, and we spent time looking for generic and easy-to-read symbols. The signage is implemented in both our dementia units and our general nursing units within our homes to help with continuity during the transition for residents who may have lived in other communities in other parts of the home previously. The signs can be installed on the doors of the day areas but if the doors are most often held open, they can also be wall mounted.

We install bathroom signage on all bath/shower rooms, and also all toilets, including en-suites, as we refurb the home. This helps to maintain continuity within the community and helps residents to recognise a familiar symbol. The signage for back-of-house areas (such as the clinical room) are installed at the top of the doors, and therefore out of the residents' line of sight.

Toilets and bathrooms

Good design mixed with good functionality in our bathroom areas has been one of our main points of focus. We want our interiors to provide a pleasurable experience for the resident but also to help to promote good continence and personal hygiene.

Making bathrooms identifiable in a corridor full of doors is one of the most important aspects of design in enabling residents to live as independently as they can within their environment. Bathroom doors of a different hue and tone to the rest of the corridor also help them stand out. During our pilot we wanted to trial a colour that to us seemed an obvious bathroom-related colour: a blue tone, but also one that had a light reflectance value differential that falls within the regulations specified in the Disability Discrimination Act (DDA) and BS8300 that relate to enhancing an individual's spatial awareness to help them use their residual vision to navigate. The implementation of this has so far had success, with some residents who previously were unable to find the toilet independently now being able to visit the toilet alone. The colour chosen is well liked by residents and families alike and also looks smart and calming within our environments.

Within the bathrooms themselves it is all about visual accuracy and recognition: the key elements need to stand out to enable residents with vision impairments to identify the correct sanitaryware. The method we have introduced as a visual aid is to use a contrast tile behind the toilet and hand wash basin in all wash areas and en-suites. This generally includes using a darker tile all around the bottom of the toilet area, but if carrying out a small refurb, contrasting tiles could be used behind the toilet and wash-basin. The tiles of choice are fresh and contemporary, and using a darker tile behind the crucial bathroom elements enables them to stand out but retain a homely feel, as traditional and familiar designs will help to ease anxiety and help promote self-care (King's Fund 2014). With this in mind, we also decided to utilise a traditional tap design similar to those that the resident may have used in their previous home, as the look and feel of the taps is familiar and easy to use. The hot and cold symbols are obvious; the design is simple and streamlined. To aid with recognition, these taps are utilised in all basins across the board, including assisted toilets and en-suites.

An internet search of terms such as 'dementia bathroom designs' or 'dementia-friendly bathrooms' will provide numerous examples of bathrooms designed to enable care home residents with dementia.

Rest areas

Areas where residents can sit and relax in corridors and in smaller lounge spaces are extremely important for their safety and well-being (King's Fund 2014). We have created small break-out spaces, which have softer lighting and a stronger colour on the walls to create a relaxing and restful space for people to sit in to take a break whilst travelling around the home. The photographic murals also take pride of place in these locations, in calm, serene images in soft colour tones, which transport the viewer to a peaceful mindset. These areas play a large part in the health and safety aspect of our corridors, but also are a much-visited quiet destination for residents and families alike. A recent report has highlighted that, for some people, different realities created by others could cause more confusion and distress but in our experience, the rest areas (with photographic murals) have provided much comfort for those who choose to sit and reside in them (Williamson and Kirtley 2016).

Lighting

Most importantly, sufficient lighting has been shown to be a central aspect of a supportive environment (Noell-Waggoner 2002). Sufficient lighting is a prerequisite for successful navigation and good vision; it helps the resident perceive the shape and size of corridors and rooms but also observe cues for orientation. We ensure all our installed lighting is now energy-efficient LED as there were lots of problems associated with the older fluorescent lighting, such as flickering bulbs and a low-level humming sound.

The lighting levels need to be high and to almost emulate a bright sunny day. The lighting is at the same level throughout the corridors and we utilise a recessed faceted down-light style, which bounces the light level out in an even, balanced and consistent way. The illumination disperses evenly across the spaces, reducing the risk of any shadows that, unfortunately, residents can interpret as holes to step over. We removed the wall lights in corridors, as these were a distraction for residents and also created shadows on the walls. Ceiling lighting not only enables the fittings to blend into the background but also creates a more natural style of illumination. Lighting surveys and good design ensure we have the correct levels of lux (amount of illumination provided) for the vision of our residents.

Several studies have focused on the positive effects of artificial bright light, including increased sleep duration and less aggressive and agitated behaviour (Calkins *et al.* 2007).

Carpet and flooring

Installing the right texture, aesthetic and colour underfoot can make a critical difference to the health, well-being and day-to-day life of someone living with dementia. The flooring makes a difference to the transition around the building as people with dementia might perceive dark patterns or decisive separations of one area from another as three-dimensional, and be afraid of the 'steps' or 'holes' in the floor (Namazi *et al.* 1989; Passini *et al.* 2000). With this in mind, and also with our own experience of working alongside residents with dementia, we took a different approach to the specification. We wanted a floor covering which would promote a calm environment and be a colour that would blend in well with the surroundings. The decision to go with the majority of flooring as carpet has many benefits; research has shown that carpets are associated with the lowest number of fractures per 100 falls, as the mean impact is significantly lower on carpeted floors (Simpson *et al.* 2004). Carpet also helps with sound absorption and keeping a peaceful atmosphere. We decided on a neutral mid-tone colour scheme, which promotes a feeling of calm, serenity and tranquillity. The tone of the carpet blends in with our palette of schemes and provides a great platform for any interior co-ordination. The colour also matches in with the en-suite and dining flooring which therefore enables us to utilise the colour throughout the unit from the bedrooms, down the corridors and into the day rooms. Visually this helps the resident move around the unit safely, without causing any hesitation from the appearance of a step or a hole. The benefits of this flooring are not only creating a safer environment for our residents, to reduce the risk of falls, but also using a colour of carpet that blends into the background, allowing the residents to observe more around them, such as the signage for the toilet or artwork to trigger a memory. The carpet is plain with no flecks or pattern, which therefore reduces the risk of distraction for the resident or danger of throwing them off balance.

The dining areas required a flooring that harmonised well with the carpet choice to avoid the visual 'step' but also that emulated more of a domestic environment and homely ambiance. We chose a natural wood-effect style, without too much of a defined grain or texture to it. Visually it merges in with the carpet, but it also exudes a calming and familiar atmosphere and undertone.

Summary

This may seem to be an odd chapter to put into a book looking at activity in dementia care but we thought it was important to highlight that the environment has had a huge impact in some of our homes where we have introduced the new key concepts. Many of our residents enjoy spending their days walking around, and whilst they do not seem anxious (or looking for a way out), we wanted to provide some form of activity or engagement on their travels. In addition, if people feel less anxious about where they are, they are more likely to be involved in 'everyday home life' within the care home. We have certainly seen fewer incidents of distress within the homes, and we feel that a large part of this is due to the residents feeling less frustrated as the changes have helped them to find their way around and, perhaps most importantly, to their own rooms. Relatives have also commented that the themes and pictures within the corridors have provided them with a source of 'conversation' or activity with their resident.

Five key points for consideration

- The use of colour and themes can help residents to independently navigate their way around the home.

- Themes and pictures can provide stimulation for residents who wish to walk around, or 'talking points' for staff as they walk around with the resident.

- Rest areas can help residents who choose to walk around to take a break.

- Signage is really important and should be clear and have both visual pictures and written words.

- The environment should be as 'homely' as possible to encourage the residents to relax and engage in activity when they choose.

10

Summary

CAROLINE BAKER

Keeping occupied and stimulated can improve quality of life for the person with dementia, as well as for those around them. Activities can act as an opportunity for fun and playfulness. They can also encourage independence, social inclusion, communication or expression of feelings (Alzheimer's Society 2016).

The level of activity or engagement that a resident wishes to participate in is almost as unique as their fingerprint, inasmuch as everybody has their own beliefs, wishes and 'fun' levels that may change on a daily basis depending upon their mood. The key to us providing meaningful activity or engagement for the residents in our care is for us to really get to know the resident and their usual preference for involvement. Another of our skills is to read the signs when it is apparent that the resident would rather not be involved in anything and simply chooses to relax and watch the world go by.

We have had some surprising results with some of the activities that we have tried and tested, particularly with the use of empathy dolls and the digital show reels: residents who we were not sure would respond well to these interventions exceeded our expectations and either became fully engaged or demonstrated an increase in their well-being levels.

The activity interventions were part of a wider programme that provided four levels of training (aligned to the *Skills for Care Dementia Framework* (Skills for Care n.d.)) and dementia specialist support, and which required staff to implement a number of criteria based on evidence and research in dementia care practice. Other activities were also 'tried and tested' but proved not to be so easy to implement at this time.

Musical playlists

One of our dementia care specialists brought some MP3 players and headphones for one of the homes to enable the residents to listen to a playlist of their choice. In principle, this idea is fabulous, and we have seen videos on the internet where the effect has been truly remarkable, but unfortunately on the whole it proved quite difficult to obtain the requisite media for the residents. For the few residents where we were able to establish their favourite songs, they really enjoyed listening to the music, and for some it provoked an emotional reaction, but some of our residents unfortunately did not have relatives who were able to help us and may have been unable to recall their favourite songs themselves. However, we will try again! We are very fortunate with the organisation to have a number of music therapists (one of whom has just been awarded an MBE!) who may help us to drive this innovation forward.

Intergenerational activity with the school

We also tried a fun physical activity in partnership with the local senior school. The students who were involved in the programme were given an introduction to dementia care and person-centred care and how they might communicate effectively with a person living with dementia. The students were really keen to be involved and quickly adapted to work alongside the person living with dementia. However, the activity involved the residents having to be ready at a given time, then boarding a minibus and going to the school.

For some it was quite disorientating and it was felt that the residents felt under pressure to be ready for a set time. But the residents really seemed to enjoy it whilst they were there and those not directly involved (and waiting their turn) appeared to enjoy watching the others play and listening to the fun and laughter. Going forward, the staff have suggested that the activity may be more manageable and meaningful to the residents if it were held within the care home itself.

iPad reminiscence

We worked with a company that was relatively new to the iPad world of reminiscence and unfortunately there were teething problems on both sides. Although the designated homes to trial the iPads had wireless connectivity, this was occasionally hit and miss, depending upon where the resident was within the home. In addition, some of the components of the iPad reminiscence programme did not function as well as they should and staff found it quite difficult to help the residents to navigate around the functions. In the future, we think this will be a remarkable addition to assist with reminiscence as it gives both opportunities to discover the residents' own photos and documents and also the ability to explore other avenues which may lead on, for example, to helping the residents to search for colleagues who they worked with or finding pictures of their hobbies.

Reminiscence newspaper

Three of the homes tried this intervention which involved a reminiscence-type newspaper being delivered to the home's email inbox and then a monthly round-up accompanied by a music playlist of songs that had featured within it. The intervention was successful in one of the homes which accommodated people in the earlier stage of their dementia (a residential home) but was not as successful in the homes that provided care for people with moderate to advanced dementia.

Signs of success

We have not carried out a formalised research project (although we have obtained measures on clinical data) but we know from qualitative feedback that most of the activities that we have introduced have been received really well, not only by residents but also by relatives and staff. We would like to share with you some of the comments or feedback that we have received.

Improving activity focus

> *There are more activities, such as the Memory Lane tea parties. Those are going down really well. We do them once a month. There's musical entertainment; we give everyone straw hats to wear...everyone's absolutely buzzing about it.*

> *The rummage boxes are great for going through with people who are feeling stressed. The MP3 players are great too. We create individual playlists by finding out from the residents and their families what music they like.*

> *I think activities are better when they are less institutionalised, when there are things happening all the time. I like to have activity tables with lots of things around like beach bags hanging up and picnic baskets people can rummage through. It's lovely to walk in and see people sitting around a table, engaged in something or listening to music.*

Reducing distress and improving well-being

The dementia unit is like a different place now. The residents are happy and there are very few visible signs of distress. When I go to the unit I get lovely hugs and kisses. It's my place of retreat when I'm feeling stressed. (Home that used Namaste Care as an intervention.)

The dolls work well with the residents because they look really real. They stroke their hair and look at it all – the hands and feet. They fiddle with it and look at it as if to say, 'Who are you?' I even thought they were real!

As a whole it was noticeable that people were being supported in a more person-centred way, but specifically about the management of one particular resident with regard to their restlessness and positively engaging with activities.

Residents are eating more and putting on weight, which is great to see. We have a really good chef now who has been here for a few months. Staff also always eat with residents, which makes it more social and encourages people to eat more.

Changing minds and cultures

We have a senior carer who has been here for years who used to be very task-orientated. She has made the biggest change. Now she organises nearly all the activities and she's a 10-60-06 champion. The first time she started putting it into practice, she couldn't believe the difference it made. She organises one-to-one activities and engages others in the home. For example, she engages the maintenance team by getting them to paint a box in the garden with a resident who likes that activity. She also gets outside groups to come into the home.

It has been interesting trying to get the families involved with the life story books. Some are enthusiastic and some were less positive because they thought it would be distressing to rake up old memories. It has been surprising to learn what people did in their earlier years.

The future is bright

We now have themed corridors – very colourful. Before 10-60-06 the corridors were very institutional and not specifically tailored towards people living with dementia. Now there is nice paint and the signs on room doors have been changed. The old ones had room for photos but the new ones look very neat and clean.

I think one of the biggest differences is that it's now so much brighter. There are loads of different themes: a gardening theme, beach theme, 1950s theme and a TV with a USB in it playing music and showing images from previous decades.

The environmental changes that have had the biggest impact are the new signage on bedroom doors and in communal areas, and also the use of pastel colours and the redeveloped central garden, which now has flower baskets, windmills, lots of things that make it a much nicer space for residents. The work on the garden is ongoing.

Motivating staff

The impact on staff has been great, and the training has given them increased knowledge and flexibility in their approach. They are more confident doing activities, which is great for residents because they in turn get more stimulation.

It has made a big difference to the carers, who used to say
'Activities aren't our job' but now get more involved.

Where to now?

Due (not only) to the success of the programme but also the evolving changes within dementia care and the varying needs of those living with dementia, we are continuing to evaluate, develop and roll out this programme to all of our Memory Lane Communities. We appreciate and understand the need for a programme that not only incorporates existing evidence-based best practices that enhance the lives of those we care for, but also allows for a fluid approach to new research emerging that is proven to be of benefit.

A duty of care is a requirement for all those who provide care services (and rightly so), and with this in mind we believe that it would be wrong to sit still and not regularly review the programme to ensure it meets the needs of both current and future recipients. By doing so, we believe we will always be providing the best individualised approaches whilst promoting growth and fun and recognising and promoting the voices of those whom we care for.

How can we live in a world of hope, alternatives, growth and possibility, when dementia threatens our sense of self? We need to create a new image of who we are and who we are becoming. How we do this depends very much on our personality, our life story, our health, our spirituality, and our social environment.

Bryden (2005)

References

Allen, C.K., Earhart, C.A. and Blue, T. (1992) *Occupational Therapy Treatment Goals for the Physically and Cognitively Disabled*. Rockville, MD: American Occupational Therapy Association.

Alzheimer's Society (2007) *Home from Home*. London: Alzheimer's Society.

Alzheimer's Society (2012) *The Later Stages*. London: Alzheimer's Society.

Alzheimer's Society (2014) *Factsheet: Exercise and Physical Activity*. Available at www.alzheimers.org.uk/factsheet/529 (accessed May 2017).

Alzheimer's Society (2016) News article. Available at www. alzheimers. org.uk/info/20029/daily_living/15/exercise_and_physical_activity/2 (accessed December 2016).

Alzheimer's Society (2017) *Staying Involved and Active*. Available at www.alzheimers.org.uk/site/scripts/documents_info.php?doc umentID=115 (accessed January 2017).

Apted, T., Kay, J. and Quigley, A. (2006) 'Tabletop sharing of digital photographs for the elderly.' In *CHI '06: Proceedings of the SIGCHI Conference on Human Factors in Computing Systems*. New York: ACM.

Baker, C. (2015) *Developing Excellent Care for People Living with Dementia in Care Homes*. London: Jessica Kingsley Publishers.

Ballard, C. (2016) 'Which activities are most engaging for people with dementia living in care homes?' *Alzheimer's Society, Research e-journal 11*, 4–7.

Baum, C., Edwards, D.F. and Morrow-Howell, N. (1993) 'Identification and measurement of productive behaviours in senile dementia of the Alzheimer type.' *Gerontologist 33*, 3, 403–408.

Beck, K.C. (1998) 'Psychosocial and behavioral interventions for Alzheimer's disease patients and their families.' *American Journal of Geriatric Psychology 6*, 2 (Suppl. 1), S41–S48.

British Medical Journal (2014) 'The health benefits of physical activity: Depression, anxiety, sleep, and dementia.' Available at http://learning.bmj.com/learning/module-intro/.html?locale=en_GB&moduleId=10052400& (accessed December 2016).

Brooker, D. (2007) *Person-Centred Dementia Care: Making Services Better.* London: Jessica Kingsley Publishers.

Bruce, E. (2000) 'Looking after well-being: A tool for evaluation.' *Journal of Dementia Care 8,* 6, Jan/Feb.

Bruneau, T. (1989) 'Empathy and listening: A conceptual review of theoretical directions.' *Journal of the International Listening Association 3,* 1–20.

Bryden, C. (2005) *Dancing with Dementia: My Story of Living Positively with Dementia.* London: Jessica Kingsley Publishers.

Bryden, C. (2016) *Nothing About Us, Without Us!* London: Jessica Kingsley Publishers.

Calkins, M., Szmerekovsky, J.G. and Biddle, S. (2007) 'Effect of increased time spent outdoors on individuals with dementia residing in nursing homes.' *Journal of Housing for the Elderly 21,* 3–4, 211–228.

Cayton, H. (2001) *From Childhood to Childhood? Autonomy, Dignity and Dependence Through the Ages of Life.* Available at www.alz.co.uk/adi/pdf/hcayton_childhood.pdf (accessed November 2016).

Chang, E. and Johnson, A. (2012) 'Challenges in Advanced Dementia.' In E. Chang and A. Johnson (eds) *Contemporary and Innovative Practice in Palliative Care.* Croatia: In Tech.

Damianakis, T., Crete-Nishihata, M., Smith, K.L., Baecker, R.M. and Marziali, E. (2010) 'The psychosocial impact of multimedia biographies on persons with cognitive impairments.' *Gerontologist 50,* 1, 23–35.

Day, K., Carreon, D. and Stump, C. (2000) 'The therapeutic design of environments for people with dementia: A review of the empirical research.' *Gerontologist 40,* 4, 397–416.

Dean, R., Proudfoot, R. and Lindesay, J. (1993) 'The Quality of Interaction Schedule (QUIS): Development, reliability and use in the evaluation of two domus units.' *International Journal of Geriatric Psychiatry 8,* 819–826.

Dementia Care Australia (2017) 'Activities and therapies.' Available at www.dementiacareaustralia.com/index.php?option=com_content&task=view&id=342&Itemid=75 (accessed May 2017).

Department of Health (2009) *Living Well with Dementia: A National Dementia Strategy*. London: Department of Health Publications.

Department of Health (2012) *Prime Minister's Challenge on Dementia: Delivering Major Improvements in Dementia Care and Research by 2015*. London: Department of Health Publications.

Department of Health (2015) *Policy Paper: 2010 to 2015 Government Policy: Dementia*. Available at www.gov.uk/government/publications/2010-to-2015-government-policy-dementia/2010-to-2015-government-policy-dementia (accessed April 2017).

Department of Health (2016) *Prime Minister's Challenge on Dementia 2020: Implementation Plan*. London: Department of Health.

Dow, B. (2011) 'Evaluation of Alzheimer's Australia Vic Memory Lane Cafés.' *Cambridge Core 23*, 2, 246–255. Available at www.cambridge.org/core/journals/international-psychogeriatrics/article/div-classtitleevaluation-of-alzheimerandaposs-australia-vic-memory-lane-cafesdiv/4388ABDCA5106C1C391F2C142434B817 (accessed December 2016).

Duffin, C. (2012) 'How Namaste principles improve residents' lives.' *Nursing Older People 24*, 6, 14–17.

English Oxford Living Dictionaries (2016) 'Empathy.' Oxford: Oxford University Press. Available at https://en.oxforddictionaries.com/definition/empathy (accessed December 2016).

Erskine, R.G., Moursund, J.P. and Trautmann, R.L. (1999) *Beyond Empathy: A Therapy of Contact in Relationship*. New York: Routledge.

Feil, N. (2015) *V/F Validation: The Feil Method: How to Help Disorientated Old-Old* (3rd edition). Cleveland, OH: Edward Feil Productions.

Free Dictionary, The (2016) 'Exercise.' Available at http://medical-dictionary.thefreedictionary.com/physical+exercise (accessed April 2017).

Gard, T., Holzel, B.K. and Lazar, S.W. (2014) 'The potential effects of meditation on age-related cognitive decline: A systematic review.' *Annals of the New York Academy of Science 1307*, 89–103.

Gowans, G., Dye, R., Alm, N., Vaughan, P., Astell, A. and Ellis, M. (2007) 'Designing the interface between dementia patients, caregivers and computer-based intervention.' *Design Journal 10*, 1, 12–23.

Gridley, K., Brooks, J., Birks, Y., Baxter, K. *et al.* (2015) *Life Story Work in Dementia Care.* University of York, Social Policy Research Unit. Available at http://eprints.whiterose.ac.uk/95286/1/Life_Story_Work_in_Dementia_Care_SPRU_Research_Findings_Feb_2016.pdf (accessed October 2016).

ImaginationGYM (2016) *The Enchanted Forest CD and Activity Book Pack.* Dublin: BrightChild Productions Ltd. Available at http://store.imaginationgym.com/default.asp (accessed April 2017).

James, I., Mackenzie, L. and Mukaetova-Ladinska, E. (2006) 'Doll use in care homes for people with dementia.' *International Journal of Geriatric Psychiatry 21*, 11, 1093–1098.

Jones, G. and Miesen, B. (1996) *Care-Giving in Dementia, Volume 1.* London: Routledge.

Jones, G. and Redwood, K. (2010) *Introductory Information Pack: To Help Set Up and Host an Alzheimer Café.* United Kingdom.

Kemsley, J. (2016) 'Sixty-four per cent of people living with dementia feel isolated following a diagnosis.' *Health and Social Care Bulletin.* Available at http://ageactionalliance.org/wordpress/wp-content/uploads/2016/04/April-20162.pdf (accessed May 2017).

King's Fund (2014) *Is Your Care Home Dementia Friendly? EHE Environmental Assessment Tool* (2nd edition). London: King's Fund.

Kitwood, T. (1997) *Dementia Reconsidered: The Person Comes First.* Buckingham: Open University Press.

Kovach, C. (1997) *Late-Stage Dementia Care: A Basic Guide.* Washington, DC: Taylor & Francis.

Larouche, E., Hudon, C. and Goulet, S. (2015) 'Potential benefits of mindfulness-based interventions in mild cognitive impairment and Alzheimer's disease: An interdisciplinary perspective.' *Behavioural Brain Research 276*, 1 January, 199–212. Available at www.sciencedirect.com/science/article/pii/S0166432814003611 (accessed April 2017).

Mackenzie, L., James, I., Morse, R., Mukaetova-Ladinska, E. and Reichelt, F.K. (2006) 'A pilot study on the use of dolls for people with dementia.' *Age and Ageing 35*, 4, 441–444.

Marquardt, G. (2011) 'Wayfinding for people with dementia: The role of architectural design.' *Herd 4*, 2, 22–41.

Maslow, A.H. (1954) *Motivation and Personality.* New York: Harper.

McArdle, R. (2016) '"Keep on movin": Physical activity in dementia.' *PLoS ECR Community*. Available at http://blogs.plos.org/thestudentblog/2016/06/07/keep-on-movin-physical-activity-in-dementia (accessed December 2016).

Mitchell, G. (2016) *Doll Therapy in Dementia Care: Evidence and Practice*. London: Jessica Kingsley Publishers.

Moss, A.S., Wintering, N., Roggenkamp, H., Khalsa, D.S. *et al.* (2012) 'Effects of an 8-week meditation program on mood and anxiety in patients with memory loss.' *Journal of Alternative and Complementary Medicine 18*, 1, 48–53. Available at http://online.liebertpub.com/doi/abs/10.1089/acm.2011.0051 (accessed April 2017).

Namazi, K. and Johnson, B. (1991) 'Physical environment cues to reduce the problems of incontinence in Alzheimer's disease units.' *American Journal of Alzheimer's Care and Related Disorders and Research 6*, 6, 22–28.

Namazi, K., Rosner, T. and Calkins, M. (1989) 'Visual barriers to prevent ambulatory Alzheimer's patients from exiting through an emergency door.' *Gerontologist, 29*, 5, 699–702.

Napp Pharmaceuticals (2014) *Pain in People with Dementia: A Silent Tragedy*. London: Napp Pharmaceuticals Ltd.

National Institute on Aging at NIH (2016) 'Go4Life: 4 types of exercise.' Available at https://go4life.nia.nih.gov/4-types-exercise (accessed December 2016).

NICE (2013) *Dementia: Support in Health and Social Care (Quality Standard 1)*. London: NICE. Available at www.nice.org.uk/guidance/QS1 (accessed December 2016).

Noell-Waggoner, E. (2002) 'Light: An essential intervention for Alzheimer's disease.' *Alzheimer's Care Quarterly 3*, 4, 343–352.

Online Oxford English Dictionary (OED) (2016) Web link. Available at www.oed.com (accessed November 2016).

Oxford Learner's Dictionaries (2017) 'Activity.' Available at www.oxfordlearnersdictionaries.com/definition/english/activity?q=activity (accessed May 2017).

Passini, R., Pigot, H., Rainville, C. and Tetreault, M.H. (2000) 'Way-finding in a nursing home for advanced dementia of the Alzheimer's type.' *Environment and Behaviour 32*, 5, 684–710.

Perrin, T., May., H. and Anderson, E. (2008) *Wellbeing in Dementia: An Occupational Approach for Therapist and Carers.* Philadelphia, PA: Churchill Livingstone.

Pool, J. (2008a) *The Pool Activity Level (PAL): Instrument for Occupational Profiling.* London: Jessica Kingsley Publishers.

Pool, J. (2008b) Pool Activity Level (PAL). Available at www.jackiepoolassociates.org (accessed April 2017).

Pool, J. (2012) *The Pool Activity Level (PAL): Instrument for Occupational Profiling.* London: Jessica Kingsley Publishers.

Power, G.A. (2014) *Dementia Beyond Disease: Enhancing Well-Being.* Baltimore, MD: Health Professional Press.

Salari, S. (2002) 'Intergenerational partnerships in adult day centres: Importance of age-appropriate environments and behaviours.' *Gerontologist 42,* 321–333.

Shattell, M.M., Starr, S.S. and Thomas, S.P. (2007) '"Take my hand, help me out": Mental health service recipients' experience of the therapeutic relationship.' *International Journal of Mental Health, 16,* 274–284.

Simard, J. (2013) *The End-of-Life Namaste Care Program for People with Dementia* (2nd edition). Baltimore, MD: Health Professional Press.

Simard, J. and Volicer, I. (2010) 'Effects of Namaste Care on residents who do not benefit from usual activities.' *American Journal of Alzheimer's Disease and Other Dementias 25,* 1, 46–50.

Simpson, H.H., Lamb, S., Roberts, P.J., Gardner, T.N. and Evans, J.G. (2004) 'Does the type of flooring affect the risk of hip fracture?'. *Age and Ageing 33,* 3, 242–246.

Skills for Care (n.d.) 'Endorsement framework.' Available at www.skillsforcare.org.uk/Learning-development/Endorsement-framework/Endorsement-framework.aspx (accessed May 2017).

Stacpoole, M., Hockley, J., Thompsell, A., Simard, J. and Volicer, L. (2015) 'The Namaste Care programme can reduce behavioural symptoms in care home residents with advanced dementia.' *International Journal of Geriatric Psychiatry 30,* 702–709.

St Christopher's Hospice (2014) 'Namaste Care programme: Making life meaningful for people with very advanced dementia.' Available at www.stchristophers.org.uk/care-homes/research/namaste (accessed July 2017).

Stokes, G. (2004) 'A Person-Centred Understanding.' In G. Stokes and F. Goudie (eds) *The Essential Dementia Care Handbook*. Bicester: Speechmark Editions.

Su, T.W., Wu, L.L. and Lin, C.P. (2012) 'The prevalence of dementia and depression in Taiwanese institutionalized leprosy patients, and the effectiveness evaluation of reminiscence therapy – a longitudinal, single-blind, randomized control study.' *International Journal of Geriatric Psychology 27*, 2, 187–196.

Swaffer, K. (2016) *What the Hell Happened to My Brain? Living Beyond Dementia*. London: Jessica Kingsley Publishers.

Tang, Y., Hölzel, B.K. and Posner, M.I. (2015) 'The neuroscience of mindfulness meditation.' *Nature Reviews Neuroscience 16*, 213–225. Available at www.nature.com/nrn/journal/v16/n4/abs/nrn3916.html (accessed April 2017).

Tilly, J. and Reed, P. (2008) 'Literature review: Intervention research on caring for people with dementia in assisted living and nursing homes.' *Alzheimer's Care Today 1*, 24–32.

Toms, G.R., Clare, L., Nixon, J. and Quinn, C. (2015) 'A systematic narrative review of support groups for people with dementia.' *International Psychogeriatrics 27*, 9, 1439–1465.

Trueland, J. (2012) 'Soothing the senses.' *Nursing Standard 26*, 43, 21–22.

van Alphen, H.J., Volkers, K.M., Blankevoort, C.G., Scherder, E.J., Hortobágyi, T. and van Heuvelen, M.J. (2016) 'Older adults with dementia are sedentary for most of the day.' *PLoS ONE 11*, 3. Available at http://journals.plos.org/plosone/article?id=10.1371/journal.pone.0152457 (accessed April 2017).

Williamson, T. and Kirtley, A. (2016) *Dementia Truth Inquiry: Review of Evidence*. London: Mental Health Foundation.

Xiong, G. and Doraiswamy, P.M. (2009) 'Does meditation enhance cognition and brain plasticity?' *Annals of the New York Academy of Science 1172*, 63–69.

Subject Index

Author Index

Allen, C.K. 66
Alzheimer's Society 65, 67, 119, 183
Anderson, E. 71
Apted, T. 50

Baker, C. 27, 28, 66, 161
Ballard, C. 66
Baum, C. 71
Beck, K.C. 49
Blue, T. 66
British Medical Journal (BMJ) 117
Brooker, D. 102, 156
Bruce, E. 72
Bruneau, T. 67
Bryden, C. 23, 31, 36, 37, 103, 189

Calkins, M. 180
Carreon, D. 51
Cayton, H. 86
Chang, E. 66

Damianakis, T. 59
Day, K. 51
Dean, R. 69
Dementia Care Australia 165
Department of Health (DOH) 22, 103, 106
Doraiswamy, P.M. 141, 142
Dow, B. 103
Duffin, C. 64

Earhart, C.A. 66
Edwards, D.F. 71
English Oxford Living Dictionaries 89
Erskine, R.G. 65

Feil, N. 94
Free Dictionary 117

Gard, T. 141
Goulet, S. 142
Gowans, G. 50
Gridley, K. 40

Holzel, B.K. 141
Hölzel, B.K. 142
Huson, C. 142

James, I. 86
Johnson, A. 66
Johnson, B. 174
Jones, G. 27, 102

Kay, J. 50
Kemsley, J. 103
King's Fund 172, 175, 177, 178, 179
Kirtley, A. 179
Kitwood, T. 55, 91, 98
Kovach, C. 70